A Clinician's Guide to Methamphetamine

A Clinician's Guide to Methamphetamine

Jeanne L. Obert, M.F.T., M.S.M.

Michael J. McCann, M.A.

Patricia Marinelli-Casey, Ph.D.

Richard A. Rawson, Ph.D.

HAZELDEN®

Hazelden
Center City, Minnesota 55012-0176

1-800-328-9000
1-651-213-4590 (Fax)
www.hazelden.org

ISBN-13: 978-1-59285-183-6

Library of Congress Cataloging-in-Publication Data

A clinician's guide to methamphetamine/Jeanne L. Obert … [et al.].
p. ; cm. — (Hazelden professional library)
Includes bibliographical references.
ISBN 1-59285-183-5 (pbk.)
1. Methamphetamine abuse. 2. Methamphetamine. 3. Amphetamine abuse. 4. Drug abuse. I. Obert, Jeanne L. II. Hazelden Foundation. III. Series.
[DNLM: 1. Amphetamine-Related Disorders—therapy. 2. Methamphetamine. WM 275 C641 2004]
RC568.A45C55 2004
362.29'9—dc22

2004059941

09 08 07 06 05   6 5 4 3 2 1

Cover design by David Spohn
Interior design and typesetting by Kinne Design

CONTENTS

ACKNOWLEDGMENTS

This *Clinician's Guide to Methamphetamine* contains information gathered by the authors during the past twenty years. During most of this time period, medical care for the Matrix Institute was overseen by our close and valued colleague, Walter Ling, M.D. Besides the names mentioned here, there have been many others who have actively participated in developing the Matrix experience for meth users. While there are too many to mention, a few deserve special recognition.

For about fifteen years, Paul Brethen, M.F.T., directed the Matrix office in Rancho Cucamonga. As a result, he has probably served as therapist for or overseen the treatment of thousands of meth users. He made the Rancho Cucamonga Matrix office into a valuable part of the San Bernardino County Health Department service delivery system and the Rancho Cucamonga community. Don Smith, M.S., and Alan Mann, M.F.T., set the office up, and William Shalhoub, M.S., provided the initial funding for the office. As the meth epidemic has spread in the greater Los Angeles area, meth users have entered treatment provided by Matrix at other clinic sites. Andrea Weiner, Al Hasson, Sam Minsky, Greg Allen, Leana Gadbois-Sills, Deborah Service, Dan George, and Janice Stimson have been among the key managers at Matrix and have administered, delivered, or supervised the care of thousands of meth and cocaine users. Finally, during the twenty years of the Matrix organization, more than three hundred marriage and family therapists, psychologists, interns, and trainees have delivered service to drug- and alcohol-dependent individuals and their families. Although they are not listed here by name, we would like to thank all of these people for their contribution to the Matrix organization and to the care of its patients.

PREFACE

by Richard A. Rawson

In the mid-1980s, large numbers of methamphetamine (meth) users began to seek treatment in some parts of California, Hawaii, and other western states. One such area was San Bernardino County, California. Several communities in western San Bernardino had long been the home of some of the largest organized groups of motorcycle gangs. For these groups, meth production and sale were among the main sources of revenue. As a result, meth was widely available and very inexpensive in the surrounding communities. Unfortunately, during the last twenty years the meth situation in this part of California has not improved, and the damage done to the users, their families, and communities has spread throughout much of the United States and many other parts of the world.

When meth users sought substance abuse treatment in the 1980s, they found the system offered several major forms of treatment, but none of the treatments suited their needs. For example, twenty-eight-day inpatient programs, designed to treat alcoholics, were expensive and not accessible to many of the users who did not have medical insurance. Outpatient methadone maintenance programs were clinically/medically inappropriate for treating people with stimulant use disorders. Long-term therapeutic community programs, with residential treatment plans of six to twelve months, were viewed by many meth users and their families as impractical and unacceptable, since meth users often were employed and had family and financial responsibilities. In many instances, Alcoholics Anonymous members were not receptive to the needs of younger "tweakers" whose addiction experiences were quite different from those of the older alcoholics.

At this point in history, the objectives of outpatient substance abuse treatment (excluding methadone maintenance programs) weren't clearly defined. There were no established treatment protocols, and the rationale, content, duration, and intensity of most treatment programs were entirely idiosyncratic. Meth users entering outpatient treatment could receive anything ranging from a weekly group session to intensive treatment of three hours per day for five days. In many places, the treatment approach was an adaptation of inpatient or residential treatment materials. There was little, if any, data on the efficacy or effectiveness of such treatment programs for meth users.

The Matrix Organization

In 1984, three of the authors of this guide (Richard Rawson, Jeanne Obert, and Michael McCann) established the Matrix Organization (and were soon joined by Patricia Marinelli-Casey) with the expressed purpose of developing treatment protocols for outpatient substance abuse treatment and employing principles and techniques supported by empirical evidence. Matrix's goal was to create treatment protocols that would meet the specific needs of cocaine and meth users. In the first Matrix office, in Beverly Hills, California, the vast majority of patients were cocaine users, with an occasional gay male meth user from Hollywood/West Hollywood. The second office, opened in 1986 in Rancho Cucamonga, California, was situated at "ground zero" of the meth epidemic. The treatment and research teams in the Rancho office have produced much of our clinical experience and research data on meth. Since 1986, approximately ten thousand meth users have been treated here. It is from these patients that we have learned about meth use and recovery.

The Matrix Model

The Matrix Model *Intensive Outpatient Alcohol and Drug Treatment* is a comprehensive, evidence-based, sixteen-week individualized program with more than twenty years of research and development by the Matrix Institute on Addictions, an affiliate of the University of California at Los Angeles (UCLA) Integrated Substance Abuse Programs (ISAP). This treatment curriculum was published by Hazelden in 2005.

The mission of the Matrix Institute on Addictions, a nonprofit organization, is to improve the lives of individuals and families affected by alcohol and other drug use through treatment, education and training, and research by promoting a greater understanding of addiction disorders. Matrix Institute's primary goal is to improve the quality and availability of addiction treatment services. The focus of the Institute is to disseminate accurate, empirically based information in the health care system.

Matrix clinics in the greater Los Angeles area serve as sites for many service projects administrated by the institute as well as research studies conducted by the UCLA Integrated Substance Abuse Programs. The projects conducted at the clinics carefully study the elements that produce addiction and promote recovery so that we can better understand the processes of addiction and recovery. Conducting this research and disseminating the findings to the widest possible audience are the primary goals of the institute. Matrix staff have published extensive information and conduct widespread trainings on a number of subjects regarding chemical dependency treatment.

INTRODUCTION

by Richard A. Rawson

"Speed kills" was a slogan attributed to the Haight Asbury Clinic in San Francisco during the late 1960s. The impetus for this slogan was that when amphetamine made its entry into the "flower power" drug culture of the Haight, people started dying. Although the pharmaceutical amphetamine (the "speed" of the 1960s) is no longer available, the use of one form of amphetamine, methamphetamine (meth), has clearly reached epidemic proportions in much of the United States. Meth use is the dominant drug problem in the western and midwestern portions of the country, most severely affecting rural areas. Recently, rates of meth use have risen sharply in some East Coast cities among gay men. Meth is a central nervous system stimulant that produces intoxication through the increased stimulation of dopamine and norepinephrine receptors in the brain. The alertness, euphoria, and sense of well-being that result from the use of meth last considerably longer (eight to twelve hours) than similar effects resulting from cocaine use (one to two hours), and the drug is metabolized by the body at a much slower rate.

How to Use This Guide

This clinician's guide is designed for practitioners who encounter meth users in treatment. It is intended to provide clinicians with knowledge about meth abuse and dependence and some strategies that may help in the treatment of meth users. In working with these patients, it is important to know what the drug does to the body and the brain and how people addicted and in recovery feel, think, and behave. The information on treatment is based on the treatment approach used at the Matrix Institute on Addictions outpatient clinics in Southern California, which has been used with more than ten thousand cocaine and meth users at the Matrix clinics as well as with thousands of others at treatment centers throughout the United States. The Matrix materials have been translated into eight languages and are used to treat meth users around the world.

What to Expect

As you will learn in chapter 1, Methamphetamine 101: The Basics, meth can be injected, smoked, snorted, or ingested orally. The timing and intensity of the "rush" that accompanies the use of meth, which results from high levels of dopamine being released into the brain, depends in part on the method of administration. Prolonged use of meth may lead to tolerance for the drug and increased use at higher dosage levels, creating a very severe dependence. Chronic use of the drug, with little or no sleep, leads to an extremely irritable and paranoid state. Discontinuing the use of meth often results in extreme depression, as well as fatigue, anergia, and cognitive impairment that lasts anywhere from two days to two weeks.

Chapter 2, Clinical Challenges in Treating Meth Abusers, covers the challenges a clinician should expect to encounter when treating meth users. Although people start using meth for a variety of psychological and sociological reasons, once it has been administered to the human brain, profound changes begin to occur. Meth appears to damage neurons in ways that are different from, and in some ways more severe than, other drugs of abuse. High dosages of meth permanently damage neuron terminals, though some regrowth may occur. Recent research at UCLA has linked chronic meth use to a very substantial reduction in the volume and functioning of important areas of the brain that control cognition, memory, and emotion. These issues provide, to say the least, some real clinical challenges.

Chapter 2 also explores the five stages of recovery for meth users (withdrawal, honeymoon, the Wall, adjustment, and resolution stages) and why it's crucial that patients know what to expect during treatment. Meth will be revealed as the true equal opportunity drug. Its price and accessibility add to its appeal. It is inexpensive relative to other illicit drugs, and it is easy to produce from commonly available chemicals. Women use it to reduce fatigue, suppress their appetites, and temporarily relieve symptoms of depression. Adolescent girls are largely attracted to it because of its weight-loss potential. Gay men find it appealing because it initially enhances sexual activities. This chapter also discusses psychiatric symptoms associated with meth, including depression, suicidal ideation, paranoia, hallucinations, psychotic reactions, panic disorders, and violent behavior. Information on medication is also provided. Currently, there is no effective pharmacological treatment available for meth dependence, but research is being conducted on several medications.

Effective treatment strategies developed by the Methamphetamine Interagency Task Force (MITF) are examined in chapter 3, Effective Treatment—It Can Happen: Combining Knowledge, Experience, and Wisdom. The task force was formed in 1996 to address the growing meth epidemic. The result: seven key strategies for outpatient treatment for meth users. Relapse prevention is an intricate part of these strategies.

Data on effective treatments for meth dependence is limited. Behavior and cognitive behavioral strategies, along with participation in self-help activities, appear to provide the most positive outcomes. One intensive, integrated outpatient approach, the Matrix Model, has been found to successfully engage meth users in treatment and result in substantial reductions in meth use. The Matrix Model *Intensive Outpatient Alcohol and Drug Treatment,* published by Hazelden, is a comprehensive, evidence-based, sixteen-week individualized program with more than twenty years of research and development by the Matrix Institute on Addictions, an affiliate of the UCLA Integrated Substance Abuse Programs (ISAP).

Chapter 4, Assessment: Getting It Right, highlights issues of particular importance to clinicians faced with properly assessing meth users. Typical areas of assessment include demographic characteristics, drug use history and diagnosis, treatment history, and other life domain problems. Although general treatment guidelines do not always call for an assessment of physical and medical functioning, such an assessment is vital with meth users due to the severity and prevalence of adverse physical health effects related to meth use. The assessment of past and present drug use is vital to treatment planning. Understanding the client's pattern of use and vulnerability to relapse are important factors when tailoring a treatment plan to best fit the client's needs.

Chapter 5, Adolescents and Meth, looks at how adolescents are getting hooked on meth and describes methods for successful treatment. Risk and protective factors of adolescents along with the three stages of adolescent substance abuse (experimental or early use, regular use, and psychological and physical dependence) are explored here. The MITF recommendations are outlined, with discussion on what they mean to adolescents in treatment for meth use.

Chapter 6, Children and Meth, is the final chapter. The negative consequences of meth don't just affect the user. Children of meth abusers are at high risk of neglect and abuse, and pregnant women's use of meth can cause growth retardation, premature birth, and developmental disorders in neonates. In addition, evidence suggests that prenatal exposure to meth may lead to cognitive problems in young children. The reported number of children present at seized meth labs across the United States has increased dramatically. Increased meth use and home-based production is linked with an escalation of reported serious child abuse and neglect. Children living in meth labs are at extremely high risk for poisoning, homicides, and accidental deaths and burns due to fires and explosions.

■ ■ ■

CHAPTER ONE

METHAMPHETAMINE 101: THE BASICS

by Michael J. McCann

This chapter explains methamphetamine (meth) basics, including how it's made, its history, the lure, and why it has become an epidemic. The chapter also describes the short- and long-term effects of the drug and how it compares to other drugs such as cocaine.

Meth Basics

Meth is an odorless, bitter-tasting crystalline powder that can be white, yellow, or brown. It is referred to as "meth," "speed," "crystal meth," "crystal," "crank," "chalk," "ice," "glass," and "tina." It can be smoked, snorted, injected, or swallowed. While it is similar to amphetamine in its chemical structure and effects, the stimulant effects are more powerful. It is defined by the *DSM-IV* as a schedule II stimulant, meaning it has a high abuse potential and if prescribed, the prescription cannot be refilled. The medical uses for meth are limited to narcolepsy (uncontrolled lapses into unconsciousness), attention deficit disorder, and obesity.

Meth is typically not acquired from pharmacies; instead, it is made in illegal labs and sold "on the street." Meth is manufactured from basic ingredients that are easily accessible, including ephedrine or pseudoephedrine, acetone, paint thinner, anhydrous ammonia, lye, and hydrochloric acid. In addition to the damage meth inflicts on those who use it, its manufacturing harms the environment. According to the Office of National Drug Control Policy, the production of one pound of meth creates five to seven pounds of toxic waste. It is not uncommon for poisonous waste products to be discarded into drains, into sewers, or simply on the open ground. Lab explosions are also not uncommon. According to the Drug Enforcement Administration, in 2001 there were 12,715 meth lab incidents reported in forty-six states. The highest rate of these occurred in Missouri, with 2,207 incidents, followed by California with 1,847 and Washington with 1,477.

History of Meth

Amphetamine was synthesized in 1887 by a German chemist, and the derivative, methamphetamine, was synthesized in Japan in 1893. It was initially used in nasal decongestants and inhalers. Meth use was not common until World War II, when it was used to increase endurance (e.g., for pilots on long missions). Following the war, widespread use of meth occurred in Japan and has continued to the present day. In the United States in the 1960s, amphetamines were prescribed for weight control and depression, with thirty-one million prescriptions written in 1967 alone. Following greater controls on prescriptions for amphetamines and methamphetamine, illicit meth labs materialized. Until relatively recently, meth use had been associated primarily with West Coast biker gangs and long-distance truck drivers. Today, it has expanded to white-collar workers, students, minorities, and women.

The Meth Epidemic

Meth use has spread over the past decade to epidemic proportions. Meth use is a particularly dominant drug problem in the western and, more recently, midwestern and Appalachian regions of the United States, most severely affecting rural areas. In some areas, such as San Diego County, San Bernardino (California) County, and Honolulu, meth use has continued without interruption through the 1980s to the present. In other parts of the West and Midwest, use erupted in the late 1990s and has since spread rapidly.

The Substance Abuse and Mental Health Services Administration (SAMHSA) reports that the proportion of meth users seeking treatment (out of all substance abuse treatment admissions in the United States) increased from 1 percent in 1992 to 6 percent in 2001. In thirty-three states, the rates have at least doubled between 1992 and 2001. Emergency room visits related to meth use increased 54 percent between 1995 and 2002, according to the Drug Abuse Warning Network, with increases in the West, Midwest, South, and Northeast. These trends will likely continue, considering that the National Survey on Drug Use and Health reported an increase of more than 100 percent in the number of people who have tried meth between 1991 and 1998.

Internationally, meth use is second only to cannabis in terms of the percentage of the population reporting past-year use, with ranges significantly higher in Thailand, Honduras, Philippines, Ireland, Australia, and New Zealand. It is estimated that 10 percent of people in substance abuse treatment worldwide are seeking help for a meth problem. According to the World Health Organization, more than thirty-five million people regularly use or abuse amphetamine/methamphetamine. By contrast, cocaine use is limited to approximately fifteen million people worldwide (mostly in North America), and heroin is used by fewer than ten million people.

Factors Contributing to the Epidemic

Without question, epidemics of illicit drug use in American society have shown a cyclic pattern, with heroin, cocaine, meth, hallucinogens, and marijuana trading places as the "drug du jour." However, over the past fifty years it has become apparent that heroin, cocaine, and marijuana have escalated from periodic flare-up usage to ongoing endemic problems. The use of heroin, even with variations in purity, is a constant in major U.S. communities. In the 1980s, cocaine use also became an epidemic. Although its use among people in the middle class has dramatically decreased since 1994, the use of crack cocaine is still the single biggest blight on many large inner-city communities. Marijuana use clearly is not a transient phenomenon. Use among teens shows periodic increases and decreases, but few drug abuse experts expect that marijuana use will disappear.

There have been two notable instances of drug epidemics that appear to have come and gone since the mid-1950s without becoming severe problems. Hallucinogens, including LSD, psilocybin, and mescaline, gained major public attention in the late 1960s and early 1970s. The popularity of these powerful psychedelics—boosted by rock musicians and such widely read authors as Timothy Leary and Carlos Castaneda—created near social hysteria about their dangers. According to virtually all drug use indicators, use of hallucinogens since the 1980s has decreased to a very low level. Similarly, the use of phencyclidine (PCP) in some parts of the country during the late 1970s created very significant concerns among health care and law enforcement officials. However, whether supplanted by the cocaine epidemic of the 1980s or simply losing momentum on its own, the PCP scare was for the most part a short-lived epidemic.

Will the meth problem continue as a significant health and law enforcement concern? Or will it go the way of acid and PCP and be of interest only to a few devotees and drug abuse historians? While there is no way of predicting with certainty the future course of this meth epidemic, the following reasons suggest it will not end soon.

Ingredients Are Easy to Find

Obtaining the ingredients to make meth is relatively easy. Most of them can be found at your local hardware store. While international efforts to eradicate coca production and prevent coca importation might someday reduce cocaine supplies, availability of the ingredients needed for meth production cannot feasibly be eliminated.

It's Inexpensive

Meth is likely to remain available and inexpensive as well. Meth effects are long lasting (eight to twelve hours), and users typically spend about one-fourth as much for meth as cocaine users do for cocaine.

It's Easy to Make

Since 1994, knowledge of how to manufacture meth has been disseminated from a few "biker gang cookers" to two very important new groups: "mom-and-pop chemists" and organized drug trafficking cartels. With the addition of these two groups, the availability of meth is likely to increase as new markets are created. Creative mom-and-pop chemists can now print meth recipes from the Internet and produce small quantities for personal and associates' use.

It's Appealing

Many users are initially attracted to meth for two reasons: it helps reduce fatigue and aids in weight reduction. It is possible for people to use meth for years before intolerable negative consequences occur. Under these "controlled use" circumstances, the user maintains functioning longer than with other "less controlled" patterns of use. For example, they "hit bottom" more slowly than heroin users (who have the severe consequence of opiate withdrawal to motivate treatment entry) or cocaine users (who experience profound losses due to the costly and uncontrolled binge pattern of smoked cocaine). "Controlled use" makes meth seductive and usually ends in addiction.

Meth—Whom It Affects

Historically, meth use has been linked to specific groups (such as bikers) and geographic areas (the West, Northwest, and Hawaii). With the continuing spread of meth use, new groups have been affected, including those living in rural areas, gay and bisexual men, students, workers, adolescents, women, and children.

Those Living in Rural Areas

The strong odors (similar to cat urine, ether, or ammonia) given off by labs have made rural areas well suited for meth production. As a result, Nebraska, Iowa, Wyoming, Colorado, Missouri, and other areas not typically associated with severe drug problems have huge meth problems.

Gay and Bisexual Men

The rate of meth use among gay and bisexual males is alarming. Many meth users combine the drug with sexual activities, finding that it extends and intensifies their sexual experience. For some men, the association between meth and sex becomes so strong that it is difficult to have sex without using drugs or experiencing severe drug cravings. Other men are reluctant to abstain totally from meth because it reduces their inhibitions and allows for episodes of sexual behavior that would be unlikely without the drug's use.

Meth use may lead many gay and bisexual men to engage in risky sexual behaviors. Because meth is associated with sexual expression, it is often used in bathhouses and sex clubs to enhance sexual encounters. Under the influence of meth, many men may have unprotected sex, possibly with multiple partners. Unprotected anal intercourse places these men at risk for HIV and other infectious diseases. While many men (including heterosexual men) use meth to enhance their sexual experiences, long-term use and high doses are often associated with impotence and sexual dysfunction.

Students

Many meth users can sustain their ability to function and work for long periods of time—a fact that is appealing to students. Meth use has been reported among young athletes, cheerleaders, models, medical students, and beauty pageant contestants. In a substantial number of anecdotal reports, high-achieving students have relied on meth to help them maintain both their good grades and an active social schedule.

Workers

Meth use in the workplace is on the rise, as people look for ways to sustain their ability to function and work for long periods of time. According to Quest Diagnostics, the incidence of meth-positive urine tests in the workplace increased 68 percent from 2002 to 2003. Eventually, productivity suffers as the meth user becomes dependent on the drug and can no longer concentrate.

Adolescents

Illicit drug use by adolescents, who are still developing physically and emotionally, is a serious concern. It may affect their ability to make decisions, interfere with their social development, and result in injuries and accidents. Research indicates that meth use may permanently change parts of the brain.

One recent study of adolescents entering substance abuse treatment found that females were using meth at higher rates than their male counterparts. Another study by the National Center on Addiction and Substance Abuse at Columbia University focused on females ages eight to twenty-two over a period of three years. This study found that girls and young women become dependent upon meth faster and suffer adverse effects sooner than boys and young men.

Women

The use of meth is more prevalent among U.S. women than is the use of any other illicit substance. Why? Some speculate that the reason is the current social demands on women, who are often expected to fulfill and excel in multiple roles. During initial use, meth provides energy, enhances self-confidence, and improves body image, leading many women to view meth as a readily available, inexpensive appetite suppressant and energy enhancer. However, users experience a crash that can cause depression, irritability, insomnia, nervousness, and paranoid and aggressive behaviors after the intense, euphoric high wears off. Over time, everyday functioning suffers as meth use leads to serious medical and psychiatric symptoms.

Children

According to both research studies and law enforcement reports, rising meth use across the United States has dramatically escalated the severity of child abuse crimes and raised the rate of child abuse homicides. The growth of home-based meth labs means that more children are being exposed to the drug and the toxic chemicals used to make it. Children can suffer poisoning, burns, and lung irritation; damage to the liver, kidneys, heart, brain, and immune system; cancers such as lymphoma and leukemia; bone marrow suppression resulting in anemia and increased risk of infections; and developmental and growth problems.

Besides being exposed to meth and its precursor chemicals, these children are often the victims of their parents' drug-focused lifestyles that many times are characterized by neglect, physical or sexual abuse, domestic violence, and other criminal activities. In addition, children of drug-dependent parents are at high risk to continue intergenerational patterns of drug abuse, criminal behaviors, and neglectful parenting.

How Is Meth Taken?

Meth can be snorted, smoked, injected, or swallowed. Approximately 60 percent of users smoke meth, 20 percent snort it, and 20 percent inject it. How it is administered affects the speed of onset, the dose delivered to the brain, and the intensity of it. It may also influence the course of abuse and the progression to dependence. Drug use traditions, culture, and geography seem to influence how it is administered. For example, injecting meth is most common in the northwestern region of the United States, while smoking meth is most predominant in Hawaii. Keep in mind that preferences in how the drug is used change over time and probably will not remain the same in the future.

Intranasal Use (Snorting)

When meth is snorted, it generally reaches the brain within three to five minutes, although the "high" may not be perceived as immediate. The drug's effects can last from eight to twelve hours, depending upon the dosage, without repeated exposure. Potential adverse reactions to intranasal use include sinusitis, loss of the sense of smell, congestion, atrophy of nasal mucosa, nosebleeds, perforation or necrosis of the nasal septus, hoarseness, problems swallowing, and throat ailments.[1]

Smoking

When smoked, meth reaches the brain within seconds and produces an almost immediate effect. But this intense high can lead to intense lows and drug cravings. Some of the medical consequences of smoking the drug include hoarseness, problems with swallowing, throat ailments, and a productive cough with black sputum.[2]

Injecting

Meth can be injected directly into the bloodstream or muscle. When users inject it into the bloodstream, the drug reaches the brain in fifteen to twenty seconds. Medical consequences associated with intravenous use or the sharing of contaminated drug paraphernalia include HIV, hepatitis, tuberculosis, lung infections, pneumonia, air bubbles that stop the heart, wound abscesses, blood clots, kidney failure, and vein inflammation.[3] Injection drug users should be immediately referred to a physician to be checked for infectious diseases and other medical complications resulting from injection use that may include sharing dirty needles.

Both drugs and alcohol have immediate and long-term physical and psychological effects. The user typically seeks the immediate psychological effect of euphoria and sometimes other immediate effects such as tranquilization, alertness, or a sense of confidence. The inability to control the drug or alcohol use brings the long-term effects into the picture. As meth use increases and moves into dependency, the immediate effects may still be experienced, but there is a preponderance of the negative long-term effects as well.

Swallowing

Meth reaches the brain about twenty to thirty minutes after being swallowed in pill form. Users often place it in a mixed drink to dissolve. In pill form, the drug is absorbed more slowly by the body. The effects are less extreme when meth is swallowed, but last longer (up to twelve hours).

Meth Effects

Meth affects the brain almost immediately, increasing dopamine and producing a feeling of euphoria. Dopamine is a neurotransmitter associated with pleasure both through natural rewards (food, water, sex) and through activation by cocaine and meth. Cocaine also causes increases in dopamine, but meth use results in brain damage not seen from cocaine or other drug use.

Meth use compromises normal brain functioning. In animals, evidence of damage to brain cells has been found after a single high dose, and continued changes in the brain can be detected for many months. Scientists have found that after discontinuation of the drug for one year, meth users still exhibit changes in the brain associated with motor and cognitive impairments. These changes were found in people who had used for less than one year.

Dr. Paul Thompson of UCLA described "a forest fire of brain damage" in a brain mapping study of meth users that he conducted. He found an 11 percent loss in tissue in the brain's pleasure/reward centers in meth users in their thirties who had used for ten years. The Partnership for Drug Free America's 1987 portrayal of fried eggs as "your brain on drugs" was dismissed by many as on over-the-top scare tactic. While this is up for debate, a twenty-first-century version of "your brain on drugs" could replace fried eggs with brain scans of meth users and would factually represent what the eggs attempted only symbolically.

Meth, along with alcohol and other drugs, has immediate and long-term psychological and physical effects. People use in order to experience the immediate effects, but as use becomes uncontollable, the long-term, negative effects increase.

Meth's Immediate Effects

Immediate psychological effects are

- euphoria
- increased alertness
- increased confidence

Immediate physical effects are

- dopamine release in the brain
- increased heart rate
- increased blood pressure
- increased respiration
- tremors
- pupil dilation
- increased sex drive
- decreased fatigue
- decreased appetite

Snapshot of the meth user:

After taking meth, the user usually appears alert, talkative, and sometimes "twitchy." Actions are rapid, and thoughts can be loosely associated, resulting in a tumble of topics and ideas. A general sense of well-being is apparent.

Meth's Long-Term Effects

Long-term psychological effects are

- paranoia
- irritability
- depression
- confusion
- cognitive impairment (poor memory and thinking)
- drug cravings
- psychotic symptoms (hallucinations, paranoia, and delusions)
- suicidal thoughts

Long-term physical effects are

- tolerance (more drug is required to produce the desired effect)
- addiction
- weight loss
- damage to blood vessels in the brain and possible stroke
- fatigue
- damaged brain cells
- seizures (can be fatal)
- hyperthermia (can be fatal)

Snapshot of the meth user:

The chronic user is often emaciated and poorly groomed. Repetitive movements, nonsensical talking, extreme agitation, anger, paranoia, violence, depression, lethargy, or sleepiness are all common in the chronic user.

Meth Intoxication and Withdrawal

Meth intoxication is typically seen in those who abuse the drug or are dependent on it. However, intoxication can occur after taking a single dose. Intoxication is a direct effect of drug use. Symptoms include exaggerated drug effects such as euphoria, grandiosity, restlessness, talkativeness, and repetitive behaviors. Some users might hear, feel, and see things or people that simply aren't there. These symptoms usually diminish over a period of twenty-four to fourty-eight hours once drug use has stopped.

When meth users discontinue chronic use, they experience withdrawal that can last as long as two weeks, with aftereffects lingering several weeks longer. As opposed to opioid (drugs like heroin) withdrawal, there is no drug or medication that can reverse the withdrawal experience. Primary withdrawal characteristics are depression and extreme tiredness. Other symptoms include irritability, anxiety, and drug cravings.

The length and severity of withdrawal vary, and many meth users proceed through it with minor symptoms. However, some develop such a fear of withdrawal that they continue to use reduced amounts while enrolled in treatment in order to function. They feel that they simply cannot tolerate the withdrawal or that they will not be able to continue to function as a worker, student, or homemaker.

Comparing Meth to Cocaine

The cocaine use in our society in the 1980s and 1990s brought with it an unprecedented amount of media attention. Athletes and movie and rock stars as well as the middle class and the indigent have been affected by this drug. Powder cocaine begot crack cocaine, and things got worse. A cheap and powerful high could render people powerless after a single instance of use. After years of cocaine publicity, a new stimulant comes into the spotlight and the questions are often asked: "Is meth worse than cocaine?" "What is the difference between cocaine and meth?"

Meth and cocaine are both stimulants. They both cause higher-than-normal amounts of dopamine in the brain. They both produce dependency. They both ruin lives. The table on the following page lists other similarities and differences.

The Future of Meth

There is no reason to expect that the meth epidemic will abate at any time in the near future. It has spread worldwide and has affected areas and populations not usually associated with drug dependency. The ease of manufacturing meth, its initial "usefulness," and its low cost will most likely promote the continued spread of the drug in the United States and internationally.

As long as people work long hours in tedious, physically demanding jobs, want to lose weight, or are faced with hopeless socioeconomic circumstances, the attraction of meth is likely to remain. At present, there are few signs to suggest that the current meth epidemic will simply become an unpleasant memory, as did the hallucinogen and PCP epidemics. Neither of these drug types were inviting to new users as being socially acceptable or promoting some positive purpose and allowing the user to function normally (or supernormally). On this basis alone, meth has the ability to continue to attract new users and sustain growth despite the risks of severe psychological and physical consequences.

TABLE 1

Meth versus Cocaine

	METHAMPHETAMINE	COCAINE
Raw material	Chemicals	Plant (coca)
Manner used	Injecting, intranasal use, smoking, oral use	Injecting, intranasal use, smoking, oral use (rarely)
Duration of "high"	8–12 hours	1–2 hours
Neurotoxicity	Yes	No
Stroke risk	Yes	Yes
Psychosis, paranoia possible	Yes	Yes
Increased HIV risk behaviors	Yes	Yes
Urban use	Yes	Yes
Rural use	Yes	Minimal

■ ■ ■

CHAPTER TWO

CLINICAL CHALLENGES IN TREATING METH ABUSERS

by Patricia Marinelli-Casey

Treating methamphetamine (meth) abusers poses unique challenges for clinicians, counselors, and health care professionals. Meth's chronic effects produce medical and psychiatric symptoms that often require interventions unfamiliar to even the most seasoned substance abuse counselor. In this chapter, the early stages of recovery and the clinical features of protracted abstinence from meth will be reviewed along with medical complications of the drug, cultural practices, geographic differences, and overdose potential. The special needs of meth abusers will be highlighted along with strategies for engaging and retaining these people in treatment. The chapter concludes with information on meth-induced psychiatric symptoms and co-occurring psychiatric disorders, along with medication information.

Stages of Recovery

Meth users move through a series of stages during the recovery process. These stages appear to be based upon the brain's biological recovery after discontinuing meth use.[1]

Meth Stages of Recovery

- ***Withdrawal Stage (Day 0–Day 15)***
- ***Honeymoon Stage (Day 16–Day 45)***
- ***The Wall (Day 46–Day 120)***
- ***Adjustment Stage (Day 121–Day 180)***
- ***Resolution Stage (Day 181–Open)***

Once clients learn about the specific stages of recovery, they are often relieved. Acknowledging these stages validates the client's experience, increases the clinician's credibility, and provides a strong rationale for extended treatment involvement. The following table outlines the timetable of the stages and typical issues experienced in recovery.

TABLE 2

Meth Stages of Recovery

WITHDRAWAL STAGE (DAY 0–DAY 15)
During withdrawal, clients are disoriented, depressed, and very fatigued. They feel out of control and do not understand what is happening to them. Very explicit direction is required during this period.
HONEYMOON STAGE (DAY 16–DAY 45)
During this period, cravings are reduced, mood improves, energy increases, and confidence and optimism return. Frequently, clients feel that the problem is over and their activity becomes scattered, inefficient, and frenetic. Seeing no obvious need for continued treatment, clients may return to alcohol and secondary drug use and discontinue recovery activities.
THE WALL (DAY 46–DAY 120)
This period is viewed as the major hurdle in meth recovery. Relapse vulnerability increases as clients experience a return of low energy, little pleasure in life, difficulty concentrating, irritability, loss of sex drive, and insomnia. Clients often assume that these conditions will persist indefinitely. The Wall has also been referred to as protracted abstinence.
ADJUSTMENT STAGE (DAY 121–DAY 180)
A great feeling of accomplishment often occurs after making it past the Wall. This can result in a sense that everything should return to pretreatment normalcy. Clients who successfully deal with this stage begin to adjust to lifestyle and relationship changes, which began in previous stages, as the new definition of normal.
RESOLUTION STAGE (DAY 181–OPEN)
Completion of the six-month sobriety period signals a shift from learning new skills to monitoring for relapse signs, maintaining a balanced lifestyle, and developing new areas of interest. For some, individual or relationship issues may emerge that require additional attention.

Hitting the Wall

Of the five stages, the Wall has been described as the most difficult because it is associated with high rates of relapse and treatment termination. A common thought at this point is "If this is how I'm going to feel as a sober person, I don't think it's worth the work." The depression, low energy, insomnia, and lack of pleasure common during this period are typically not extremely severe. However, they appear endless and are often perceived by the meth user as permanent.

The following concepts are important to share with recovering people before they hit—and while they hit—the Wall:

- Remember that it takes time for your brain to heal.
- Remember that it may take time to make sense of your feelings.
- Be patient; don't give up.
- Be wary of thoughts such as, "This isn't worth it. I'm never going to feel better. I might as well use."

It has been hypothesized that the Wall is the result of a biological healing process occurring in the brain. As of this writing, it is unclear if any of the medications being evaluated for meth abuse treatment relieve these symptoms. Physical exercise does appear to alleviate the severity of the Wall. Fewer symptoms are reported by clients who exercise twenty minutes per day, three to five times per week. Continued support and encouragement by the therapist and participation in Twelve Step meetings can also be of tremendous assistance in overcoming this hurdle in the recovery process.

Overdose

Overdose and emergency treatment are common when high doses of meth are used. Overdose symptoms can include slowing of cardiac conduction, ventricular irritability, hypertensive episodes, hyperpyrexic episodes, seizures, and anorexia. Any of these symptoms warrants an immediate referral to emergency care. The Drug Abuse Warning Network reports a 61 percent increase in emergency room meth-related cases from 1996 to 2002. In 2002, 18,000 people mentioned that their emergency room visit was induced by or related to meth use (and possibly other drugs as well). Approximately 24 percent of these individuals sought medical attention due to meth overdose.[2]

Medical Evaluation

Regardless of how meth is ingested, all meth users should receive a medical evaluation prior to treatment. Meth use can produce psychosis, severe paranoia, weight loss, and other symptoms, some of which can lead to emergency situations. Clinicians treating meth users outside of a medically supervised substance abuse treatment program should be made aware of the acute and chronic effects of meth and the medical and psychiatric complications of it. Information on both the short- and long-term effects of meth can be found in chapter 1.

Special Populations and Settings

Gaining an understanding of culture, sexual orientation, geography, and circumstantial factors that affect a person's decision to enter treatment is challenging. To maximize treatment effectiveness, special consideration and sensitivity should be given to the cultures, settings, beliefs, and unique characteristics of meth users while in treatment.

Adolescents

Risk factors for adolescent substance abusers include poor family relations, parental drug use, and involvement with deviant and substance-using peer groups. School problems such as receiving failing grades, cutting class, and receiving suspensions are also related to drug use. Adolescent users are also more frequently exposed to violence and abuse (verbal, physical, and sexual). Feelings of depression and suicidal thoughts are also common, along with a history with the juvenile justice system.

An adolescent treatment plan should be based on a comprehensive assessment that includes information in the following areas: drug use history, family relations, medical complaints, psychological functioning, school performance, legal issues, and exposure to violence and abuse. Special attention should be given to the issues of weight loss, diet, and body image for females since these are often the reasons they first started using meth. See chapter 5 for more information on meth treatment specifically for adolescents.

Women

Women meth users often face both internal and external barriers that keep them from initially seeking treatment. These barriers can include guilt, shame, fear of children being taken away, fear of exposing a partner's drug use, fear of domestic violence, need for child care, lack of money, and lack of accessible treatment programs in the community. Reducing barriers is a key to engaging women in treatment. One way to do this is to provide child-care services on site. Women are also more likely to enter treatment by first having contact with other medical or social service agencies. For example, a visit to a child's pediatrician or involvement with a child protective agency may be the point of referral and entry into the substance abuse treatment system.

Treating women for meth dependence can involve a variety of issues. These include pregnancy, children, domestic violence, abuse history, parenting abilities, and socioeconomic problems. How these factors are addressed in treatment is likely to affect long-term treatment outcome.

Gay and Bisexual Men

Understanding the culture and needs of this population will improve the likelihood of a successful treatment outcome. Given the high prevalence of HIV infection, treatment for meth dependence needs to incorporate strategies that help to reduce the risk of high-risk sexual behaviors. Clinicians providing treatment for gay and bisexual men need to be aware of the powerful link between sexual behaviors and meth use and discuss it openly with their clients. A discussion of its relationship to relapse is imperative for the recovering client. In addition, clinicians must address the fears associated with the client's future sexual experiences without using meth. Many men have had few sexual encounters without the drug and are concerned about an inability to perform or the social isolation they may experience when not using. Safer sex practices and relapse scenarios that are intimately related to sexual experiences and self-confidence need to be discussed. Clinicians should feel comfortable asking questions so the client can openly discuss these topics and thereby benefit from the treatment experience.

Legally Mandated Clients

People enter the substance abuse treatment system in many ways. Some voluntarily seek help. Others are forced by family or mandated by the criminal justice system. Contrary to popular belief, it is not necessary for clients to be internally motivated to succeed in treatment. In most cases, new clients enter treatment as a result of a negative event in their lives. Because legal consequences are so easily identified, the common misconception is that progress will proceed only as long as the legal threat exists. In fact, many clients who are forced or legally mandated to enter treatment do as well or better than those who self-refer. In a multisite comparison of treatments for meth dependence, arrestees who received treatment in the context of a drug court were retained in treatment at a higher level than clients in other treatment conditions.[3] Drug court participants were required to attend treatment for eighteen months, obtain employment, clear their driving and traffic violation records, resolve other legal problems, and complete medical and psychological evaluations, as appropriate.

Legally mandated clients can be referred through the judicial system (diversion programs, California's Proposition 36, drug courts, and family drug courts), probation departments, or parole agencies. The practices and reporting requirements of these agencies and systems vary by state and by county. Some clients are eligible to receive treatment services in lieu of incarceration, depending upon the offense and prior criminal history. Others are mandated to treatment after incarceration. For clinicians unfamiliar with the criminal justice system, working with the law-involved client requires some additional education. There are often mandates for treatment that must be followed. Clients may be placed back in custody at the court's discretion if they are noncompliant with treatment or other requirements. An open relationship between the referring system, the clinician, and the client helps to develop an effective treatment plan.

Rural Populations

Meth use in rural areas has increased dramatically since 1994. Special challenges to treatment in rural areas include poverty, lack of public transportation, long commutes to reach service providers (sometimes more than one hour), limited resources, and a fragmented system of medical care and social services. In many rural communities, substance abuse treatment services are simply not available. In those that do provide services, many clinicians report feeling overwhelmed by the number of meth users seeking treatment and their lack of expertise in working with these clients. Compared to those who use alcohol and other illicit drugs, meth users may present more medical and psychiatric complications. When hospitalization or psychiatric services are needed, clinicians must make extra efforts to coordinate treatment. The issue of confidentiality and the lack of anonymity inherent in small-town life must also be considered. People may be reluctant to attend self-help meetings for fear their neighbors will find out.

Additionally, small communities often must spend large chunks of their law enforcement budgets on taking down meth labs and combating the criminal activities associated with meth use.

Psychiatric Symptoms in Meth Users

Meth use is associated with myriad psychiatric symptoms, including depression, suicidal ideation, paranoia, hallucinations, psychotic reactions, panic disorders, and violent behavior. Psychotic disorder, intoxication delirium, mood disorder, anxiety disorder, sleep disorder, and sexual dysfunction may occur in association with the use of meth. With meth use, as with any substance abuse disorder, it is often difficult to distinguish a drug-induced psychiatric symptom from a primary preexisting psychiatric condition.

Meth Psychosis

The existence of amphetamine psychosis is well documented.[4] Similar to amphetamine psychosis, meth psychosis (also known as amphetamine-induced psychotic disorder or intoxication delirium) is associated with chronic, high-dose, or continuous use of meth and produces a psychotic syndrome closely resembling paranoid schizophrenia.[5] Heightened anxiety and paranoid delusions characterize this. Auditory and visual hallucinations are common, accompanied by restlessness, agitation, and excitement. Delusions may last for a short time, though in some cases, they may endure for a longer period of time after drug use has stopped. Meth psychosis usually responds to anti-psychotic medications such as haloperidol (Haldol) and phenothiazines typically used to treat schizophrenia. The typical emergency room protocol includes haloperidol (5 mg), clonazepam (1 mg), Cogentin (1 mg), a quiet, dimly lit room, and restraints (if necessary). Someone recovering from meth psychosis may not remember it at all or remember just parts of it because of amnesia. In some cases, meth-induced psychosis may persist for several years. For some, reexposure to small doses of meth after long-term abstinence may produce paranoid psychosis.[6]

Meth-Induced Mood Disorder

A meth-induced mood disorder may occur when depressive mood features persist well beyond drug withdrawal. It is particularly difficult to distinguish a meth-induced mood disorder from a primary mood disorder, since many of the depressive symptoms are characteristic of both conditions. In addition, meth use may aggravate the intensity of a primary depressive disorder. Clinical observations suggest that antidepressant medication does not always help. Some clinicians have hypothesized that antidepressants are helpful in treating primary mood disorders but produce few beneficial effects in meth-induced mood disorders.

Meth-Induced Anxiety Disorder

Meth can induce repetitive, stereotyped behaviors similar to those seen in obsessive-compulsive disorder. It can also induce panic attacks in those with no prior history. However, it is rare for these symptoms to last beyond intoxication and withdrawal. When symptoms do persist, the person will require additional clinical attention beyond primary substance abuse treatment. Distinguishing a meth-induced anxiety disorder from a primary anxiety disorder can be difficult.

Meth-Induced Sleep Disorder

Meth can produce insomnia and sleep deprivation. During withdrawal, people may also experience hypersomnolence and nightmares. However, when these symptoms last well beyond the withdrawal period, they may require a separate diagnosis and treatment.

Meth-Induced Sexual Dysfunction

Many people use meth for the enhanced sexual experiences it provides. However, long-term use and high doses are often associated with impotence and sexual dysfunction. The relationship between meth use and sexual behavior is complex because it may produce different sexual responses depending on the stage of addiction, or different responses in men and women. For example, one study found that meth use did contribute to prolonged sex, but many study participants found that prolonged use of meth eliminated or impeded their sexual desire.

Co-occurring Psychiatric Disorders

Those with substance abuse disorders commonly experience co-occurring mental disorders. Rates for comorbidity as high as 53 percent have been reported for clients with drug (other than alcohol) disorders.[7] Comorbid mental disorders for substance abuse typically include major depression, alcoholism, and antisocial personality disorder.[8] Schizophrenia and substance abuse is also common.[9]

In a study of heroin users, higher percentages of affective and anxiety disorders were found in women than in men.[10] Although much research has been conducted on heroin, cocaine, and alcohol and their co-occurrence with psychiatric disorders, relatively little is known about co-occurring mental disorders and meth dependence. One study from Taiwan reported high psychiatric comorbidity among persons incarcerated for meth abuse, with prevalence rates of major depression (6.2 percent), alcohol use disorder (20.9 percent), pathological gambling (4.9 percent), and antisocial personality disorder (7.4 percent). All of these rates are higher than those found in the general population in Taipei. Women also reported suicidal behaviors more than men.

Treatment Considerations

It is difficult to accurately diagnose a psychiatric disorder when a meth user first enters treatment. Psychiatric symptoms do not necessarily warrant a dual diagnosis. They are often the result of meth use and subside once someone stops using the drug. Although the rates of psychiatric comorbidity are high among meth users, an accurate diagnosis requires clinical skill and sophistication. A person should have at least thirty days of abstinence from meth before a non-meth-induced psychiatric diagnosis is made. An investigation of a person's mental health history should be conducted, too. Since people with co-occurring disorders may need to receive services from more than one mental health professional or service organization, communication among such professionals is essential.

Medication

In January 2000, the National Institute on Drug Abuse (NIDA) funded a project called the Methamphetamine Clinical Trials Group (MCTG). It stimulates research to fill gaps in scientific knowledge about the pharmacology, toxicity, epidemiology, prevention, and treatment of meth abuse. Five research sites are currently conducting clinical trials, with locations in Costa Mesa, California; Des Moines, Iowa; Honolulu, Hawaii; Kansas City, Kansas; and San Diego, California. Discussions of adding new sites are underway as more cities become highly populated with meth users and inundated with meth-related problems.[11]

UCLA Integrated Substance Abuse researchers believe that in order for a medication to be beneficial in the treatment of meth abuse, it should do one or more of the following:

1. Reverse meth overdose reactions in the manner in which naloxone reverses opioid overdose reactions.

2. Alleviate symptoms of the meth "crash" in early withdrawal. Relief from the withdrawal symptoms of depression, anxiety, difficulty concentrating, and severe craving could facilitate entry into long-term and more intensive treatment.
3. Provide ongoing pharmacologic support for continued meth abstinence beyond the initial withdrawal period. This support could aid the recovery by
   - decreasing craving over an intermediate period of withdrawal in the way that nicotine gum is used in the treatment of nicotine dependence
   - satisfying meth cravings with a maintenance medication that provides a long-term substitute for meth, similar to a methadone maintenance approach to meth addiction
   - producing a pharmacologic blockade to prevent readdiction similar to the role of naltrexone in heroin addiction treatment

As of this writing, there is no effective pharmacological treatment available for meth dependence. Research is being conducted on the following medications although none has been approved by the Food and Drug Administration (FDA):

- Selegiline, the monoamine oxidase-type B (MAO-B) inhibitor
- Reserpine, the atypical neuroleptic/antihypertensive medication
- dopamine agonists (e.g., cabergoline)
- gamma-aminobutyric acid (GABA) agonists (e.g., tiagabine)
- dopamine uptake blockers (e.g., GBR 12909)
- antidepressants (e.g., bupropion and sertraline)
- 5-hydroxytryptamine (5HT3) antagonists (e.g., ondansetron)
- Ca++ channel blockers (e.g., amlodipine)

■ ■ ■

CHAPTER THREE

EFFECTIVE TREATMENT—IT CAN HAPPEN: COMBINING KNOWLEDGE, EXPERIENCE, AND WISDOM

by Jeanne L. Obert

This important chapter looks at effective treatment strategies that were developed by the Methamphetamine Interagency Task Force (MITF). This task force was established in 1996 to respond to the growing meth epidemic. The result: seven key strategies that will be outlined here on how to provide the most effective (to date) outpatient treatment for meth users.

The Meth Challenge

A frequently cited myth claims that only 5 percent of meth users can be treated successfully. No research data or other information exists to support this claim—it is simply not true. Yes, meth addiction is a challenge, but it is not untreatable. The meth epidemic has created a dilemma for some addiction treatment providers, who report that their traditional treatment programs are not effective with meth abusers. Programming does not usually provide tools to help the client deal with the powerful cravings and relapse issues unique to meth dependence. Moreover, there is limited availability of residential services, particularly for clients who do not have insurance or other resources.

Editor's Note: Over the years, it has become evident that clients who combined research-based treatment with a spiritual commitment to recovery did better maintaining long-term sobriety than those who did not. Twelve Step programs, such as Alcoholics Anonymous, have long provided a spiritual path for people desiring recovery from addictions. For that reason, the author has inserted, under chapter subtitle headings, a few Twelve Step slogans to emphasize the content. These phrases of wisdom are paired with points of information that have more recently been supported with research findings.

Outpatient treatment programs face an issue that more traditional inpatient treatment programs don't—getting each and every client to make the decision to return to the next treatment session. Research indicates that the ability to engage and retain clients in treatment is often the factor separating the effective treatment programs from those that are not. Since meth-abusing clients are particularly difficult to engage and retain, many treatment providers have concluded it is impossible to provide effective treatment. This is not the case. Although it can be challenging, it can be done. This chapter will review the specific challenges encountered and outline the key elements necessary in providing effective treatment for meth-abusing clients. First, we will review the MITF's emerging research priorities.

Meth Task Force

The Methamphetamine Interagency Task Force (MITF) was established in 1996 in response to the Comprehensive Methamphetamine Control Act and the growing problem of meth. This legislation allowed the U.S. attorney general to gather a group of experts from law enforcement, prevention, education, and treatment fields to research and report on the current efforts to combat the meth epidemic. This task force spent two years compiling a report on what prevention and treatment for meth currently looks like, what new information is available, how to use it to create future treatments, and what remains unknown. To gain the most balanced input, the task force met with both local and federal experts and attended community forum meetings. The task force recommendations included following research-based treatment principles and providing treatment as part of a comprehensive continuum of care, with proper resources and appropriately trained providers. The final MITF report, published in 2000, included the following recommendations:

- Increase the methamphetamine treatment capacity in the community and in correctional facilities.
- Increase treatment access by providing health insurance parity for substance abuse treatment.
- Increase treatment resources to address sufficiently the protracted recovery period of methamphetamine abusers in treatment. (Research suggests that methamphetamine treatment must be of a sufficient duration to address adequately the extended timetable of methamphetamine recovery.)

- Provide effective outreach services to individuals in need of treatment.
- Train and encourage mental health and medical professionals to identify and refer methamphetamine abusers to appropriate treatment settings.
- Ensure that the service delivery system includes a comprehensive continuum of care that meets the specific needs of methamphetamine abusers.
- Increase the ability of publicly funded treatment systems to respond rapidly to emerging drug problems, particularly in underserved rural areas.
- Develop methamphetamine treatment guidelines.
- Facilitate the adoption of effective research-based approaches to the treatment of methamphetamine abuse through such methods as disseminating existing research findings and training clinicians and supervisors.
- Fund and evaluate models of methamphetamine treatment that employ empirically supported treatment strategies adapted for specific high-priority target populations.
- Ensure followup services for abusers who are released from prisons and jails.
- Increase resources for drug court participation by methamphetamine abusers.

While we have made headway in the areas of prevention, education, treatment, and law enforcement on many of these recommendations, much remains to be done. Here are the research priorities set by MITF:

1. Examine existing methamphetamine prevention and education strategies that are included in broad prevention programs targeting all forms of drug use and determine the extent to which they have been effective.
2. Support research on the initiation to methamphetamine use as well as the progression of use leading to addiction.
3. Collect additional data on the extent of methamphetamine use, focusing on a number of areas (e.g., adolescent use, prevalence in rural and tribal

areas) and continue to develop and build existing databases, making them more sensitive to local communities.

The task force research recommendations have provided the basis for funding and policy decisions since 2000.

Effective Outpatient Treatment

The MITF identified seven key elements in an effective outpatient treatment program for stimulant abusers (including meth clients).

Establish a Collaborative, Positive Therapeutic Relationship

"You alone can do it, but you can't do it alone."

"When you do all the talking, you only learn what you already know."

As mentioned earlier, clients who have been abusing meth are particularly difficult to engage in the treatment process, as the continued use of stimulants, and in particular meth, leads to an extremely irritable and paranoid state when the drug use ends. Paranoia is a strong and debilitating symptom of prolonged meth abuse. In this state of mind, sitting in a crowded waiting room filling out forms becomes a scary ordeal. Clients will feel safer if they are seen by someone who understands the hallucinations and/or paranoid episodes that they may be experiencing and who can assure them that these symptoms will diminish with continued abstinence.

Though meth abusers often experience a greatly impaired memory, they are able to call up episodes of past use very quickly. Any small thing can trigger this memory. The stimulant user typically recalls a great euphoria that sets off a painful craving for the drug. These vivid memories of extreme pleasure kick the craving into a higher gear, which leaves the user reeling and feeling out of control. Treatment providers who can explain this process to the person entering treatment in a manner that reduces shame and fear have a much greater chance of establishing a trusting, nonjudgmental relationship with the client. For more information on triggers and cravings, see page 33.

There is another aspect of meth abuse that interferes with the counselor's ability to be initially helpful to the potential client. Since the drug is not viewed as being physically addictive (it does not cause a tissue dependence or obvious withdrawal), many users disassociate their addiction and other problems.

While users often feel and act very paranoid and psychotic as a result of the brain chemistry changes created by meth, they frequently do not see that these mental states are created by the drug abuse. They are unable to connect their psychiatric discomfort with their drug use. Instead, they blame the people and situations around them for their circumstances. They strongly believe that if the external situation were different, they would not need to be using the drug. To them, the very thing that is causing them problems is viewed as a solution. This situation often prevents the severely impaired meth abuser from seeking treatment. This truly is a drug of paradox.

Motivational Interviewing

Successful treatment requires a strong therapist-client relationship. The therapist's skill in engaging and retaining the client is tested on many levels. A sophisticated therapist will make it easy for the client to continue to attend the groups. The client's dignity may be very low at the treatment start, so the therapist needs to build and foster feelings of self-worth, keeping in mind that the client needs to be engaged in the recovery process for it to succeed. For this to occur, the therapist should create a safe environment where clients are treated with dignity, warmth, and respect.

Motivational interviewing is a style of client interaction developed by William Miller and Stephen Rollnick. It is designed both to enhance the therapeutic relationship and to help people become more willing to participate in the change process, to take responsibility, and to move more successfully through the stages of change as defined by James Prochaska and Carlo DiClemente. Motivational interviewing has proven successful in helping providers engage and retain drug and alcohol abusers in the outpatient treatment process. The Matrix Model of intensive outpatient treatment relates to clients in this way. In the Matrix Model, the therapist determines what approach is most likely to be effective with a particular client. The approach chosen should communicate to clients that the therapist really is interested in them as a person and truly cares about helping them help themselves. Therapists should be trained to learn how to create this change-friendly, nurturing environment.

The following example highlights how traditional and motivational interactions contrast.

TRADITIONAL INTERACTION	
Client: I just don't like going to meetings. I know it's required in this program, but they don't work for me and I'm not going to go!	***Counselor:*** You might not like it, but you have to do it or you'll be out of the program. I know that once you go a few times, you'll see the value of attending meetings, and then you'll begin doing better in treatment.
MOTIVATIONAL INTERACTION	
Client: I just don't like going to meetings. I know it's required in this program, but they don't work for me and I'm not going to go!	***Counselor:*** It seems like you feel pretty strongly about this issue. Tell me more about how you decided that meetings don't work for you.

The goal of the motivational interaction is not only to get the client to meetings but also to get the client to attend meetings with an open mind. Motivational interviewing seeks to help the client make the decision to go, rather than being forced to go and developing a resistance to participating in the Twelve Step meetings. In addition to helping the client move toward accepting what meetings have to offer, this style of interaction also increases chances that the client will feel understood by the therapist and will want to continue treatment. Learning how to interact with clients in a motivational way helps build a collaborative, positive therapeutic relationship.

Contingency Management

Research shows that contingency management (CM) is another tool to help programs attract clients and encourage participation. Providing some kind of reward for attendance, clean urines, or another identified behavior greatly stimulates continuation of that behavior. More about this important topic will be covered in the section Positively Reinforce Desired Behavior Change, page 35.

Create Explicit Structure and Expectations

> *"Ninety meetings in ninety days."*
>
> *"If you fail to plan, you plan to fail."*

The Importance of Program Structure

Creating structure is critical to the effectiveness of any outpatient program, particularly in early treatment. While inpatient programs have four walls to contain clients, outpatient programs have to teach clients how to create a structured environment within which recovery can occur. Structure is created by establishing clearly defined and predetermined activities that decrease stress and promote consistency and predictability that counter an addictive lifestyle. Structure also establishes a group norm and atmosphere that promotes the learning of new skills, such as identifying triggers and cravings. When treating meth users in an outpatient environment, learning these skills and practicing behaviors that promote safety are the first order of treatment. This is the parallel research-based intervention that is also expressed in Twelve Step terms such as "avoid slippery places and people."

One of the ways to help clients is to teach them how to schedule their time. This means actually logging in a day's activities before the day begins—either hour-by-hour or in blocks of time (e.g., morning, midday, afternoon, and evening). The intent is to change the frenetic pace of an addictive lifestyle. Clients often thrive in a protected environment where their stress level is lowered through a predictable schedule. When clients plan their time carefully, a safer lifestyle awaits them. Scheduling is also a good exercise for the brain. Planning ahead, creating an activity plan, and looking to the future allows the rational brain to function. If clients can learn to actually write down and follow a schedule each day, they will be more likely to establish a new, safer lifestyle.

The recovering stimulant user needs to be taught to predetermine activities by using the rational brain for planning. Mastering this skill is useful during both early recovery and later recovery. In later recovery, it may be necessary to go back to the basics to regain control of a relapse or to stabilize a person. Note that scheduling does not mean listing one appointment after another. Not only would this be grueling and exhausting, it would be impossible for a person to maintain. Instead, a realistic schedule, or time plan, might include activities such as taking naps, watching television, and talking with sober friends. When done properly, planning includes things that are normally part of someone's routine as well as recreational activities, exercise, attending Twelve Step meetings, and so on. When clients develop such a plan, counselors get a glimpse of what the client's life outside treatment is all about. Clients also have a chance to recognize what activities and events might prove dangerous to their recovery efforts and can schedule alternate activities. By following the schedule created with care before the day began, relapse can be avoided.

Meth and Sex

There are other qualities of this drug that make the creation of structure problematic. Many meth users associate sex with their drug use. The use of the drug extends and intensifies their sexual experience. Under the influence of meth, many engage in risky sexual behaviors such as unprotected sex, sometimes with multiple partners. In addition to greatly increasing the abuser's chance of contracting and transmitting diseases such as HIV, many users begin to associate their drug use with their sexual activity and to engage in very high-risk scenarios. As noted in chapter 2, unprotected sex in gay, urban, meth-using communities, as well as in heterosexual communities, has become a major concern in many areas. The prevalence of both the drug and the spread of communicable diseases in these communities makes the high-risk behavior especially dangerous. This behavior also makes it more difficult for clients to create and maintain structure in an outpatient treatment setting.

Provide Information and Cognitive Behavioral Concepts

> *"Don't intellectualize; utilize."*
>
> *"Change the thought and the feeling will follow."*

The U.S. government has given drug abuse research a high priority during the last several decades. Although we are learning more and more about the nature of addiction and effective treatments, this information needs to be more readily available to those who are personally fighting a battle with this disease.

When clients are educated about their addiction, they know what to expect in recovery and their treatment. Information about addiction and recovery is often an early relief to clients and their families and a client motivator. Clients often find comfort in learning that there is a science involved in addiction.

Explaining such material doesn't have to be done in a complicated manner. As strange as it sounds, complicated brain chemistry can be made easy. In a treatment episode, especially early on, the client may need the information to be short, clear, and to the point. During basic lectures, brain images can be shown to highlight the different areas of the brain affected by use. Handouts then reiterate the lesson. As the drug's effects begin to fade, clients can absorb more detailed information about their recovery process.

Including accurate, up-to-date information as part of a treatment program provides multiple benefits.

- Receiving accurate information significantly reduces the guilt and confusion that clients experience upon realizing they are addicted. Addiction is a disease comparable to any other chronic relapsing disease, such as diabetes or high blood pressure. Some of the factors that make people susceptible to this disease can also be explained. A course of treatment can be recommended that is most likely to be successful in treating the condition. When clients understand that having an addiction does not make them bad, stupid, or crazy, they are more apt to willingly enter and comply with treatment.
- Clarifying for clients why they engaged in such behaviors, while addicted, that they otherwise would never do is helpful. When people are substance dependent, they do things that they would never do drug free. The memory of that behavior is more easily forgiven if clients and their families are taught that it is not unusual to engage in addict behaviors while abusing substances.
- Educating clients that meth changes brain chemistry in a way that doesn't allow it to return to normal until almost two years following the last dose is crucial. Some studies have shown that the memory actually gets worse before it starts to recover. Stimulant abuse can cause actual structural changes to the brain, permanently damaging neuron endings. This requires a need to simplify the material. Keeping the clients informed is key to keeping them on track. See chapter 2 for a thorough explanation of the Wall stage of recovery and why it's such a stumbling block for meth users in recovery. This way, clients won't become so discouraged when they are months into their recovery and still don't feel "normal." Giving clients this information up front significantly improves their chance of achieving long-term sobriety.

- A client's future may lie in knowing that secondary drug use is the number one cause of relapse for clients dependent on stimulants. Using a secondary drug such as alcohol or marijuana first and then relapsing to meth is common. When meth addicts first enter treatment, they are often surprised to learn that the program recommends abstaining from alcohol, marijuana, and other drugs besides meth. The thinking goes something like "I came into treatment to stop using meth. Alcohol and pot are not problems for me. I don't understand why I need to stop using them." Threatening to kick clients out of treatment if they don't comply creates resistance and misses an opportunity to teach. Alternative ways to encourage compliance with this important treatment principle could include suggesting that the client not use secondary drugs for the duration of the program and delay making a decision regarding long-term abstinence until after that period. Another intervention might entail asking clients how long they could go without using pot or alcohol if they were to decide to do so and what history there is to support their belief. The ensuing discussion will result in the client talking about changing (called "change talk" in motivational interviewing), which is the first stage in actually deciding to make the change. Clients who stop using secondary drugs because they make a personal choice to do so are more likely to remain drug free after treatment than those who begrudgingly stop using because the program demands it.
- Helping addicts understand that this is not a moral issue is important, too. Once people accept that addiction is a true disease characterized by predictable behaviors and symptoms, it becomes easier to deal with the condition. Removing the stigma and shame from addiction will help clients, their families, and society at large become more effective at treating this debilitating condition. Clients and family members cannot accept the long-term lifestyle changes necessary for recovery until they understand and accept the implications of having a chronic, relapsing disease called addiction. Learning about the most recent findings on this disease provides hope and a realistic view of the recovery process.

Information: Triggers and Cravings

An important concept that explains in part the seemingly irrational and self-destructive behaviors of the meth user involves the brain and classical

(Pavlovian) conditioning. Most people are familiar with the famous "Pavlov's dog" experiment. In it, a dog hears a bell when given food. After this pairing, the bell alone will trigger salivation in the dog. A simple explanation focuses on two very powerful and different parts of the brain: the higher, rational, decision-making part; and the lower, emotional, pleasure centers. Decisions to use methamphetamine start in the higher brain as the positives and negatives associated with using are weighed. When drug use occurs, the pleasurable experiences come from the lower brain. As the negative consequences of meth use mount, users may make several decisions to stop taking the drug. But meth users find stopping to be almost impossible as cravings overpower the rational decision to stop. This happens because the people, places, and circumstances that have been associated with drug use acquire the power to trigger a response in the lower brain after a period of regular meth use. This trigger causes users to feel a craving and change their rational thinking, making use seem acceptable "one more time" or if "just a little bit" is taken. The triggered reaction in the lower brain cannot be controlled directly. This reaction is as automatic as a reflex. No number of good intentions, promises, or commitments will reduce the strength of the cravings.

Being in places or situations or around people linked with past meth use usually results in a conditioned craving and more use. The continuation of meth use despite terrible consequences is perplexing to family, friends, and even the meth user. With an understanding of the brain and the automatic, triggered cravings that result from drug use, it is easy to see why meth users cannot stop simply as a result of a decision, a promise, or the best intentions.

The information regarding this phenomenon explains past drug use and clearly indicates that the user's behavior has to change in order to avoid the triggers of cravings and establish new, healthy, and alternative behaviors. Understanding the brain and addiction makes sense out of drug-use behavior and provides the key to the first steps in recovery.

Information: Relapse Prevention

Once a period of sobriety has been achieved, the name of the game becomes relapse prevention. G. Alan Marlatt and Thomas Gordon developed the concept of relapse prevention (RP) in the mid-1980s. The concept was to teach preventive techniques to help clients recognize when they were in danger of using and how to deal with risky situations. Marlatt and Gordon also created strategies to help clients avoid a full-blown relapse if they did slip and use. Many programs, especially those delivering outpatient treatment, have adapted these easy-to-understand principles. Clients who successfully apply the principles can be quickly, easily, and positively reinforced, thereby increasing self-efficacy.

In the Matrix Model, relapse prevention techniques are taught in relapse prevention groups that meet twice a week. In each group, a relapse topic is presented both written and orally. The goal is for clients to learn new information at every meeting and to receive positive reinforcement from their therapist and other group members for sustaining their recovery. The praise delivered by peers who are further along in the process and are serving as co-leaders of each group is particularly reinforcing. In the Matrix Model, these groups are a central part of outpatient therapy.

Positively Reinforce Desired Behavior Change

"Take your body; your mind will follow."

"Fake it 'til you make it."

A successful treatment episode requires the client to absorb new information and use it to fight the addiction. Unfortunately, chronic stimulant use causes significant cognitive impairment, making treatment delivery very difficult and arduous to both the therapist and the client. Meth attacks several parts of the brain, disrupting activity and adding to the user's frustration. Stimulants greatly reduce activity in the cerebral cortex, which is invaluable in the decision-making process. This makes it difficult for the client to avoid dangerous using situations and severely impairs the ability to navigate the early stages of recovery. Without decision-making abilities, treatment becomes a real uphill battle. Making a decision to stop using is not enough to get the job done. Chronic meth use affects learning and memory, making it difficult to learn new information.

Clearly, information needs to be simplified for clients whose brains are impeded by the effects of meth abuse. Repeated failures are extremely demoralizing. Expecting the recovering person to think rationally in the face of significantly altered brain chemistry may be asking too much. Using the "one day at a time" philosophy, clients need only to follow a recovery plan that is simple, concise, and easy to understand. A supportive therapist should focus on what the client is able to do well and strongly reinforce any small step in the right direction. Goals may need to be reduced in order to help the client achieve an early win. This builds confidence and allows the episode to move in a positive direction. Therapists who are in recovery should not let their own experience or expectations for themselves drive the client's treatment.

Contingency Management

Contingency management (CM) is a powerful tool to facilitate the engagement and retention of clients in treatment and also to promote treatment progress. Rewards are made contingent upon a specified behavior, such as providing a drug-free urine sample, attending group, or achieving treatment plan goals. There is a vast research literature supporting this intervention but in treatment, CM is rarely used. The cost of CM in research studies has been high, and the methods used have been fairly complex; however, simple, inexpensive CM interventions can be used with positive results. The augmentation of traditional clinical approaches with CM can be particularly useful with meth users who may be difficult to engage and who may have difficulty with some treatment information due to cognitive impairment.

Counselors sometimes have a negative response to the notion of CM, feeling that it amounts to "bribery." Other negative feelings are often related to a belief that client motivation needs to come from within. In such cases, it may be helpful to describe CM as a motivational treatment tool to help engage and retain clients. Motivation for treatment spans a wide spectrum and many new clients are "unmotivated." With CM, these clients may avail themselves of the opportunity for treatment and give counselors a chance to help them begin the process of recovery. When used in treatment, CM provides counselors with another means of improving attendance and reducing drug use.

Most programs already have some type of reward or acknowledgment system in place. The broadening of such a system with CM use can improve treatment and raise morale at a negligible cost. Some low-cost examples of CM include

- treats provided to clients in groups
- pizza parties for clients who attend all treatment sessions or have drug-free urine tests over a specified period of time
- acknowledgements of clients who distinguish themselves (e.g., attend more than 80 percent of treatment sessions over the duration of the program; provide drug-free urine tests for thirty, sixty, or ninety days;

graduate from treatment). Acknowledgements may include a plaque, certificate, T-shirt, cap, or other item and be coupled with social reinforcement from the group or the entire clinic's staff and clients

- small gifts, trinkets, or chips to mark sobriety benchmarks (similar to those given in Twelve Step meetings)
- preferred parking or "special" seating in the waiting room or group room

Involve Family in the Recovery Process

"You are not alone."

"Active alcoholics and addicts don't have relationships; they take hostages."

In one way or another, the treatment process will affect almost everyone in the client's life. Research has consistently shown that treatment is more successful when the client's family is involved. The more family members, friends, or even work supervisors understand the process of addiction and recovery, the more supportive they can be.

Educating family members on the nature of addiction is an important first step in the process. The therapist can help family members understand why certain treatment methods are being used. Family members need to be aware that recovery is a long process involving many changes and that they need to be supportive throughout the entire treatment episode. After all, during treatment, clients will absorb a lot of information and go though many changes. Friends and family members need help in distinguishing what kind of behavior is normal and need to be prepared for the inevitable difficult periods.

Handling Strained Relationships

It is normal for clients to be reluctant about having family members involved in their treatment. At the beginning of treatment, these relationships are often strained because addictive behaviors have repeatedly caused problems. When family members have become estranged from the client, it's best to suggest that they give the person entering treatment a month or so to stabilize and prove he or she is committed to a new lifestyle. Although clients will undoubtedly struggle with the changes they must make in their lives, it is just as difficult for family members to drastically alter their behavior and attitudes.

In truth, family members need assistance in working their way through a recovery process that is parallel to that of the client. The therapist or another staff member needs to directly invite the family into this process. Clients cannot be expected to put their personal issues aside and successfully convince their alienated family members to partake in the recovery program. Families are often exhausted from enduring a long, expensive, arduous addiction and relapse process. If the addiction itself is presented as the problem—as opposed to the affected individual—the family may be more willing to participate. Even if family members do not choose to be actively involved at the outset of treatment, it should not be assumed they are forever unwilling to participate. The counselor should, with the consent of the client, continue to report progress and issue open invitations for involvement to family members. The therapist who can involve the family while maintaining a nurturing relationship with the client is building trust and optimizing the client's chance of a successful recovery.

Introduce and Encourage Self-Help Participation

> *"It works; it really does!"*
>
> *"Keep coming back!"*

Research shows a strong correlation between maintaining long-term sobriety and attending self-help groups during and after treatment. Some clients see Twelve Step programs (such as Alcoholics Anonymous and Narcotics Anonymous) and formal treatment as "either/or" options. They are not. Self-help groups and formal treatment programs can form two equally important and beneficial functions in the overall process of learning to live a drug-free life. In the United States and a growing number of other countries, these groups are widely available and free of charge. The fellowship of Alcoholics Anonymous and programs derived from it can serve many different purposes. For many, Twelve Step fellowship offers a spiritual component to recovery that is often lacking in a research-based, cognitive-behavioral treatment program.

Sober Friends = Support

Twelve Step groups also provide an opportunity to make friends with other people in recovery and to participate in drug-free activities with a group of sober people. Healthy social networks like these provide an ongoing source of support and companionship for the newly recovering person. Clients learn valuable interpersonal skills, such as how to make and be a good friend, how to persist when the going gets tough, how to forgive and live in the present, and how to deal with life on life's terms. Therapists should strongly encourage participation in these groups.

The very act of going to a meeting on a regular basis contributes to the critical structure necessary to maintain a safe and protected recovery environment. Adding self-help groups or a spiritual group that is culturally congruent to the client's recovery plan can strengthen structure. Some clients will not embrace the spiritual nature of some groups and chafe at the idea of attending additional groups. In such cases, the therapist can remind clients of the benefits of adding another recovery activity to their schedule. It makes sense for clients to use the meetings as a chance to meet people with similar problems and to put their new skills to work. It is ideal for the group to take place where the professional group meets. The convenience of this arrangement cannot be overstated, for the client is already comfortable in that setting and the other members of the group are familiar.

Use Urinalysis to Monitor Drug Use

"We are only as sick as our secrets."

"Practice rigorous honesty."

Random urine analysis (UA) is a very important part of outpatient treatment and an accurate way to monitor clients' use. These tests are not intended to bully clients or catch them in a lie about their drug use. Whether or not the therapist trusts the client is not important here. UAs should be presented in a positive light. By administering weekly drug tests, the therapist is increasing the program's structure. UAs help the therapist keep the recovery process moving in the right direction. Positive tests should not be viewed as failure but as a sign that perhaps the treatment model may need adjusting to better fit that particular client.

The clinical UA should be viewed as quite different from those done for legal reasons. However, if the client is involved in the criminal justice system, and if the on-site UAs are substituting for the legal ones, it becomes more complicated. In that case, these are not "clinical only" UAs, and they can involve a chain of custody issues, requirements to report, and so on. More information can be found in *Drug Testing in Correctional Settings: Guidelines for Effective Use* by Robert DuPont, Thomas Mieczkowski, and Richard Newel.

UAs: Standard Part of the Program

With clinical testing, positive test results may act as indicators of a problem rather than the ultimate proof of a person's sobriety. Even though positive tests carry no penalty in this clinical model, the therapist should be aware that the client may have difficulty being forthright about slips and relapses. Viewing setbacks due to relapse calmly and realistically will benefit both client and therapist. When the client has difficulty admitting use before submitting a positive test, the therapist can use this opportunity to discuss with the client what is helpful in his or her treatment plan and what may be lacking. This meeting should not be too confrontational. Instead, it can be used to provide some positive reinforcement regarding other areas of the treatment that are going well.

The addition of UAs reinforces sobriety and provides the therapist, family members, and the client with tangible proof that relapse has not occurred. Referral sources, family members, and clients entering treatment need to understand that UAs are a standard part of the program. Educating everyone involved about the important role UAs play and how the clinical UA differs from that given by the judicial system will set the stage for UA policies and procedures that benefit both the client and the program.

There Is Hope

The meth epidemic is cause for serious concern, but not reason to give up hope. Meth has a negative impact on individuals, families, and communities, but there is good news. We know that treatment for meth works. For example, a large study funded by the SAMHSA Center for Substance Abuse Treatment with almost 1,000 meth users who received either the Matrix Model treatment (a specific intensive outpatient approach) or "treatment as usual" found 60 percent meth-free at six-month follow-up.

Meth users bring some challenges to treatment, such as cognitive impairment, paranoia, domestic violence, and so on. This fact suggests that treatment modifications need to be made in substance abuse treatment. However, many of these issues are shared by alcoholics and cocaine users who have successfully completed treatment at the same programs now treating meth users. With knowledge, understanding, support, and effective treatments, there is reason for hope.

CHAPTER FOUR

ASSESSMENT: GETTING IT RIGHT

by Richard A. Rawson

Worldwide, amphetamine and methamphetamine (meth) are abused more often than cocaine. In the United States, cocaine has received greater attention due to the epidemic of the 1980s, but meth has come to represent an equally serious threat.[1] Meth has become the most popular form of amphetamine because it creates a strong high and is easy to make using readily available precursor ingredients.[2] Meth and cocaine have many similarities, including their stimulant effects on the brain and body. Yet, there are some differences between the two that should be considered when attempting to recognize and assess those with meth addiction. More information on cocaine and how it compares to meth can be found in chapter 1. This chapter will highlight issues of particular importance to clinicians who are faced with the challenge of properly assessing meth users.

Systems of Assessment—Diagnostic Categories and Criteria

Typical areas of assessment include demographic characteristics, drug use history and diagnosis, treatment history, and other life domain problems. Assessment for treatment purposes may also include consideration of socio-cultural and economic setting, family history, personal history, premorbid personality, and psychological and psychiatric disorders. Although such assessments are not always included in general drug treatment, assessing a meth user's physical health status is vital due to the severity and prevalence of meth-related physical problems.

Methods for Assessing Drug Use and Dependence

Meth use, abuse, and dependence are diagnosed with clinical tools and nonclinical assessment methods, including biological tests and self-report. Clinical tools are designed to determine whether the client meets the criteria for substance abuse or dependence. Other methods of meth assessment not intended to determine a clinical diagnosis include both objective and self-report methods. Each method has both advantages and disadvantages. For example, biological tests offer the ability to objectively ascertain use in the recent past given identified cut-off levels; however, no information about pattern, progression, and severity of use and related behaviors is possible. Conversely, self-reported use allows assessment of an unlimited amount of information about the user and his or her drug use history, but it is limited by the unknown reliability and validity of the self-reported information.

The assessment of past and present drug use is vital to treatment planning. Understanding the client's pattern of use and vulnerability to relapse are important factors when tailoring a treatment plan to best fit the needs of the client.

Diagnostic and Statistical Manual of Mental Disorders (DSM-IV)

As with other substance use disorders, the tool most often used to diagnose methamphetamine and amphetamine use disorders is the *Diagnostic and Statistical Manual of Mental Disorders.*[3] Methamphetamine-related disorders are included in the section addressing amphetamine-related disorders. Criteria for the amphetamine- and methamphetamine-related disorders of intoxication and withdrawal are presented on the next page.

TABLE 3

DSM-IV Diagnostic Criteria for Amphetamine [Methamphetamine] Intoxication

A. Recent use of amphetamine or a related substance (e.g., methylphenidate).

B. Clinically significant maladaptive behavioral or psychological changes (e.g., euphoria or affective blunting; changes in sociability; hypervigilance; interpersonal sensitivity; anxiety, tension, or anger; stereotyped behaviors; impaired judgment; or impaired social or occupational functioning) that developed during, or shortly after, use of amphetamine or a related substance.

C. Two (or more) of the following, developing during, or shortly after, use of amphetamine or a related substance:

(1) tachycardia or bradycardia [rapid or slowed heart beat]
(2) pupillary dilation
(3) elevated or lowered blood pressure
(4) perspiration or chills
(5) nausea or vomiting
(6) evidence of weight loss
(7) psychomotor agitation or retardation
(8) muscular weakness, respiratory depression, chest pain, or cardiac arrhythmias
(9) confusion, seizures, dyskinesias [impairment of voluntary movement resulting in jerky movements], dystonias [abnormal muscle tone], or coma

D. The symptoms are not due to a general medical condition and are not better accounted for by another mental disorder.

TABLE 4

DSM-IV Diagnostic Criteria for Amphetamine [Methamphetamine] Withdrawal

A. Cessation of (or reduction in) amphetamine (or a related substance) use that has been heavy and prolonged.

B. Dysphoric mood and two (or more) of the following physiological changes, developing within a few hours to several days after Criterion A:

(1) fatigue
(2) vivid, unpleasant dreams
(3) insomnia or hypersomnia
(4) increased appetite
(5) psychomotor retardation or agitation

C. The symptoms in Criterion B cause clinically significant distress or impairment in social, occupational, or other important areas of functioning.

D. The symptoms are not due to a general medical condition and are not better accounted for by another mental disorder.

Both tables reprinted with permission from the *Diagnostic and Statistical Manual of Mental Disorders,* Copyright 2000. American Psychiatric Association. Bracketed statements are additions from the author.

Amphetamine use disorders are divided into two categories based on symptomatology and severity of symptoms. *Amphetamine abuse* describes a pattern of maladaptive use of the drug leading to clinically significant impairment or distress and occurring within a twelve-month period in which the symptoms have never met the criteria for amphetamine dependence. *Amphetamine dependence,* as the more severe diagnosis of the two amphetamine/methamphetamine use disorders, is defined as a cluster of physiological, behavioral, and cognitive symptoms that, taken together, indicate that the person continues to use amphetaminelike drugs despite significant problems related to such use. Dependence is distinguished from abuse by the presence of physical factors such as tolerance and withdrawal, and by increasing loss of control over drug use.

TABLE 5

DSM-IV Criteria for Substance [Methamphetamine] Abuse

A. A maladaptive pattern of substance use leading to clinically significant impairment or distress, as manifested by one (or more) of the following, occurring within a 12-month period:

(1) recurrent substance use resulting in a failure to fulfill major role obligations at work, school, or home (e.g., repeated absences or poor work performance related to substance use; substance-related absences, suspensions, or expulsions from school; neglect of children or household)

(2) recurrent substance use in situations in which it is physically hazardous (e.g., driving an automobile or operating a machine when impaired by substance use)

(3) recurrent substance-related legal problems (e.g., arrests for substance-related disorderly conduct)

(4) continued substance use despite having persistent or recurrent social or interpersonal problems caused or exacerbated by the effects of the substance (e.g., arguments with spouse about consequences of intoxication, physical fights)

B. The symptoms have never met criteria for Substance Dependence for this class of substance.

Reprinted with permission from the *Diagnostic and Statistical Manual of Mental Disorders,* Copyright 2000. American Psychiatric Association. Bracketed statements are additions from the author.

TABLE 6

DSM-IV Criteria for Substance [Methamphetamine] Dependence

A maladaptive pattern of substance use, leading to clinically significant impairment or distress, as manifested by three (or more) of the following, occurring at any time in the same 12-month period:

(1) tolerance, as defined by either of the following:

- (a) a need for markedly increased amounts of the substance to achieve intoxication or desired effect
- (b) markedly diminished effect with continued use of the same amount of the substance

(2) withdrawal, as manifested by either of the following:

- (a) the characteristic withdrawal syndrome for the substance (refer to Criteria A and B of the criteria sets for Withdrawal from the specific substance)
- (b) the same (or closely related) substance is taken to relieve or avoid withdrawal symptoms

(3) the substance is often taken in larger amounts or over a longer period than was intended

(4) there is a persistent desire or unsuccessful efforts to cut down or control substance use

(5) a great deal of time is spent in activities necessary to obtain the substance (e.g., visiting multiple doctors or driving long distances), use the substance (e.g., chain-smoking), or recover from its effects

(6) important social, occupational, or recreational activities are given up or reduced because of substance use

(7) the substance use is continued despite knowledge of having a persistent or recurrent physical or psychological problem that is likely to have been caused or exacerbated by the substance (e.g., current cocaine use despite recognition of cocaine-induced depression, or continued drinking despite recognition that an ulcer was made worse by alcohol consumption)

Reprinted with permission from the *Diagnostic and Statistical Manual of Mental Disorders,* Copyright 2000. American Psychiatric Association. Bracketed statements are additions from the author.

Addiction Severity Index

A multitude of self-report measures exist for assessing drug and alcohol use and abuse, as well as consequences of this use; however, few meth-specific measures have been developed. Assessments of meth use typically include either a measure to ascertain a clinical diagnosis or an assessment of problematic use. The Addiction Severity Index (ASI)[4] is the most widely utilized measure for assessing problem severity in areas commonly affected by alcohol and drug misuse. These areas include medical, employment, legal, family and social support, psychiatric, and drug and alcohol use. The easy-to-administer format and its measurement of related life domains has given treatment providers a useful tool to assess clients at intake as well as throughout treatment. The ASI has been used with diverse populations, types of treatment, and drugs of abuse. It has been found to be reliable and valid in numerous settings.[5]

Biological Tests

Meth can be detected in urine for varying lengths of time—usually several days, depending on frequency of use, amount used, and sensitivity of the testing method. Metabolites can also be detected in blood, saliva, and hair. Blood and saliva furnish a better index of current levels, whereas urine provides a longer window of opportunity for detecting use. Hair analysis can reveal drug use over a period of weeks to months but has little applicability in clinical situations. Objective measures of drug use can be used alone to detect the presence of meth or to verify self-reported use. Testing biological samples for the presence of meth provides an objective measure of treatment progress. It may also help the client to resist urges and cravings by establishing accountability and reducing the likelihood of client denial.[6] Urine testing is the most common method for detecting drug use, though the less invasive technique of saliva testing is gaining in popularity.

Medical Considerations

Physical

Meth increases blood pressure and heart rate, constricts blood vessels, dilates bronchioles (breathing tubes), and increases blood sugar levels as the body prepares for the rush of the meth high, which it interprets as an emergency.

These effects can cause permanent damage to blood vessels in the brain, producing strokes, respiratory problems, irregular heartbeat, and extreme anorexia. Its use can result in cardiovascular collapse and death. Chronic meth abuse can result in inflammation of the heart lining, and among users who inject the drug, damaged blood vessels and skin abscesses. Additional dermatological problems result from repetitive, unnecessary behaviors such as skin-picking, seen with AMPH/meth drug use. Hyperthermia (elevated body temperature) and convulsions occur with meth overdoses and, if not treated immediately, can result in death.

The route of administration affects the potential for adverse reactions and associated medical disorders. Intravenous use may result in illnesses associated with the use or sharing of contaminated drug paraphernalia, including HIV and hepatitis. Taking meth intranasally can cause sinusitis, loss of sense of smell, congestion, atrophy of nasal mucosa, and nosebleeds. Meth use also leads to adverse dental effects, including unusual and accelerated patterns of dental wear due to teeth clenching and grinding. Patterns of wear are also influenced by route of administration.[7]

Neurological

Abnormal movements and facial gestures are hallmarks of chronic stimulant abuse; both acute and chronic use of AMPH and meth may result in spasmodic movements of limbs and facial muscles and uncoordination. Abnormal, involuntary movements associated with stimulant use may decrease or end when drug use is ceased; however, chronic amphetamine addicts may experience long-lasting movement disorders, persisting for several years after drug withdrawal.

Psychiatric Considerations

Psychosis

Meth use can cause a psychotic state that is virtually indistinguishable from paranoid schizophrenia,[8] and as many as two-thirds of chronic users suffer from delusional psychoses.[9] Paranoid delusions and transient auditory and visual hallucinations are frequent with this diagnosis. The delusions may be brief; however, clinicians are much more frequently reporting longer episodes, lasting several days to months.[10] Researchers have found that the severity of psychiatric symptoms strongly correlates with the duration of meth use, although psychotic symptoms have been documented in clients who have used meth for as little as three months[11] and in users as young as seventeen.[12] Although most improve with the use of neuroleptics, chronic meth users may be resistive to treatment and show continued psychotic symptoms despite extended abstinence.[13]

Cognitive Impairment

Chronic meth use may lead to cognitive impairment, including deficits in memory, problem solving, and information manipulation.[14] Adverse behavioral effects include violence and aggression, and development of stereotypical behavior patterns and repetitive behaviors that appear pointless, such as rearranging or taking objects apart.[15] Although psychological, cognitive, and behavioral functioning may return to normal after abstaining from meth for a period of time, some damage may be permanent. Appropriately assessing functioning in these areas is important in treatment efforts. Because psychological and cognitive dysfunction, such as reduced ability to process new information or make logical decisions, may interfere with the ability to benefit from treatment, it is necessary to assess psychological and cognitive functioning in the treatment setting. It is important to try to distinguish clients who *won't* from those who *can't* follow the treatment plan. Psychological and/or cognitive dysfunction may be barriers to treatment compliance, and efforts to assess and address these dysfunctions may lead to effective strategies for making improvements.

Achieving Meth Abstinence

The systematic study of factors that influence the efforts to abstain from meth use is only in its early stages. However, clinical observations do suggest that there are some issues that appear important to achieving initial abstinence from meth.

Withdrawal Discomfort

The most troublesome symptoms of the meth withdrawal syndrome are lack of energy, difficulty concentrating, and depression. These symptoms can persist for up to several weeks. Although people withdrawing from meth do not experience serious physical discomfort, their distress from the low energy and perceived inability to perform expected daily tasks can be considerable.

Frequently, after a number of days of fatigue and perceived lower-than-average functioning, cravings to use meth become very severe, which can result in relapse.

There are currently no medications that have been shown to assist people with this set of withdrawal symptoms. After long runs of meth use, in which there is substantial sleep deprivation, failure to eat, and frequently substantial musculoskeletal strain from extended drug use postures, the person is simply worn out. The needed intervention is a proper diet, rest, and exercise. Certainly, there are depletions of the neurotransmitters involved with meth effects (e.g., dopamine and serotonin); however, no pharmacological treatment strategies are currently supported by research. Many meth users are able to recover from this syndrome without medical attention. However, there are people whose psychological and physical withdrawal symptoms are so severe that they have to be temporarily housed in a drug-free environment while they achieve an initial seven- to ten-day period of abstinence. This intervention is frequently necessary with those who inject meth, who live in meth labs or with other meth users, and/or who experience severe paranoia and continuing psychotic symptoms during the early stages of recovery.

Prolonged Withdrawal

The acute meth withdrawal syndrome is readily identifiable, and the majority of symptoms are typically resolved within several days to two weeks. However, although professionals disagree about whether a true "protracted withdrawal" exists following discontinuation of meth use, many users unquestionably experience an array of symptoms that adversely affect their functioning, and these symptoms are often cited as contributing to relapse. The constellation of symptoms includes depressive symptoms, low energy, anhedonia, episodic low-grade paranoia, and various types of cognitive dysfunction. Those who suffer these symptoms generally report going through intermittent periods of days or weeks in which the symptoms are more troublesome, alternated with periods of lower severity. Recent positron emission tomography (PET) scan data[16] suggest that the entire array of symptoms represents a predictable syndrome associated with the recovery of the brain following meth discontinuation. More research is needed to explicitly define and measure the nature of this phenomenon.

Sexual Behavior

Meth users frequently associate their sexual behavior with meth use.[17] More than with other drugs of abuse, meth use very often becomes an essential and integral part of all sexual behavior for both men and women, and the meth-involved sexual activities often occur at a high frequency. This is especially true with gay men. Meth discontinuation is often associated with a decreased sex drive, ability to perform sexually, and/or pleasure derived from sexual behavior. Any or all of these sexual consequences can cause significant anxiety during the initial four to six months of abstinence. Restriction of sexual activities to avoid high-risk situations (user friends/sexual partners, gay bars, and so on) can be viewed as a tremendous sacrifice for the newly abstinent. Reduction in sex drive and/or inability to achieve an erection or reach orgasm are all viewed as catastrophic events and are frequently cited as reasons for return to use. Educating patients about the inevitable adjustment in sexual activity that occurs with meth discontinuation and pointing out that many of these negative effects are transitory can help relieve anxiety and prevent relapse.

CHAPTER FIVE

ADOLESCENTS AND METH

by Jeanne L. Obert

This chapter discusses why adolescents are getting hooked on meth and how they can be treated. It looks at the risk and protective factors of adolescents, along with stages of adolescent substance abuse. The Methamphetamine Interagency Task Force (MITF) recommendations will also be explored, taking into consideration what they mean to adolescents in treatment for meth use.

Meth use is rapidly increasing among adolescent drug users. In a July 2004 Drug Abuse Warning Network press release, the national Substance Abuse and Mental Health Services Administration (SAMHSA) reported drug-abuse-related amphetamine/methamphetamine emergency department visits increased 54 percent from 1995 to 2002. Visits involving patients ages six to seventeen increased 88 percent during the same period of time.

There is little information available about meth use in adolescents in the United States today. Part of the problem is that good systems aren't in place to gather data, although they are improving. In addition, the field of adolescent treatment is in its infancy. We are just beginning to recognize that adolescents need treatment that is different from what is offered to adults. The most reliable information about the number of adolescents using meth today was gathered through household interviews by SAMHSA's National Survey on Drug Use and Health, formerly known as the National Household Survey on Drug Abuse. It can be found at www.drugabusestatistics.samhsa.gov. Another resource is Monitoring the Future, an ongoing survey funded by the National Institute on Drug Abuse (NIDA) that was conducted by the University of Michigan. It can be found at www.monitoringthefuture.org. It reported that while past-year meth use stood at 2.3 percent of twelfth graders in 1997, that figure rose to 13 percent in 2003. Studies have shown that meth use has severe medical consequences, such as cognitive impairment, psychological dysfunction, psychopathic tendencies (auditory hallucinations), and suicidal impulses. While the specific effects on adolescents are not yet well studied, there is reason to believe that meth has serious potential morbidity in this age group.

Risk and Protective Factors

Why do some adolescents end up having problems with drug and alcohol use and others do not? The field of drug abuse prevention has spent several decades studying this issue. Several factors appear to put young people *at risk* for future drug use. Other situations seem to create protective factors, guarding against adolescent drug abuse. According to NIDA's booklet *Drug Use Among Children and Adolescents,* the following early development factors increase the risk of future adolescent drug abuse:

- chaotic home environments, particularly in which parents abuse substances or suffer from mental illnesses
- ineffective parenting, especially with children with difficult temperaments and conduct disorders
- lack of mutual attachments and nurturing

Outside the family, factors that place adolescents at high risk deal with the way children relate to school, peers, and the community. These factors include

- inappropriate, shy, and aggressive behavior in the classroom
- failure in school performance
- affiliations with deviant peers or peers around deviant behaviors
- perceptions of approval of drug-using behaviors in the school, peer, and community environments

Many of these qualities are evident in the families of adolescents who eventually find their way into adolescent treatment programs. Often the adolescent entering a drug treatment program is in need of *habilitation*, a much more difficult endeavor than the *rehabilitation* efforts common in adult programs. A recent study, in fact, showed that adolescent meth users were more likely to report greater levels of psychological dysfunction, including depression, auditory hallucinations, and suicidal ideation than non-meth users.

Young meth users also report more exposure to violence, abuse, and school and legal problems than adolescents entering treatment for other drugs of abuse.

The prevention field has also identified specific protective factors that are not just opposites of the risk factors. The strongest protective factors include

- strong family bonds
- parental monitoring with clear rules of conduct within the family unit and involvement of parents in the lives of their children
- success in school performance
- strong bonds with prosocial institutions, such as the family, school, and religious organizations
- adoption of conventional norms about drug use

The availability of drugs, trafficking patterns, and beliefs that drug use is generally tolerated influence whether an adolescent will begin using drugs.

According to statistics, many adolescents entering treatment for meth used alcohol and marijuana before moving on to meth. When protective factors are lacking, the drug has great appeal. It is a powerful stimulant that can be used when finishing a project, studying for a test, or getting relief from external pressures. At first, this inexpensive and readily available drug can be used regularly in a seemingly safe and effective way for all those purposes. The user often doesn't recognize that the drug is becoming problematic. The resulting depression, anxiety, and irritability create the need to increase the use of meth.

Meth—An Equal Opportunity Drug

Meth is the first *equal opportunity* illicit drug. Females are reporting use and for the first time are entering treatment centers in numbers equal to males. Usually, males outnumber females almost four to one. Meth gives a person more energy and, at the same time, diminishes appetite, thereby facilitating weight loss. This is often appealing for teenage girls, who feel they can accomplish more and look better. As an added bonus, it enhances sexual activity—especially for their male partners. For all these reasons, many teenage girls are willing to spin the roulette wheel and risk a serious addiction.

Much more information is still needed about this drug. This includes how to stop meth use by adolescents before it starts, what constitutes the progression of use, and more data on the motivations, risk factors, and attitudes specific to meth use by adolescents today.

Adolescents and Drug Use

While the problem severity continuum of substance use is similar for adults and adolescents, young people's drug use cannot be easily categorized using traditional criteria. Experimentation is normal for adolescents, yet the potential damage to minds and bodies in early development is significant. Therefore, many people consider any use of meth by a young person to be "abuse." Ken Winters, Ph.D., of the University of Minnesota, has identified other significant limitations of traditional diagnostic criteria when applied to adolescents:

1. Diagnostic symptoms ignore reasons for drug use.
2. Excessive heterogeneity is produced when one symptom is used to diagnose the severity of use.
3. The usual pattern of abuse leading to dependence does not always occur in adolescents.
4. A large number of adolescents who use regularly and heavily and report some dependence symptoms do not report any abuse symptoms. Because of this, they do not meet criteria for any substance use disorder.[1]

This observation further supports the importance of varying treatment interventions for adolescents along a continuum that corresponds to the severity of use by each person.

Stages of Adolescent Substance Abuse

Adolescent substance use can be conceptualized as progressing through three overlapping stages: (1) experimental or early use, (2) regular use, and (3) psychological and physical dependence. These stages are defined below along with appropriate interventions for each stage.

Stage 1: Experimental or Early Use

During this stage of drug and alcohol use, adolescents generally associate their use of substances with pleasure and mild euphoria, not negative thoughts. Most people go through this stage with no long-term consequences and do not develop compulsive habits. In fact, this type of experimental use in today's society is quite prevalent and normal. Studies have actually shown that kids who progress normally through this stage tend to be psychologically healthier, in the long term, than those adolescents who do not experience a period of experimentation or abuse.

General prevention is the treatment approach used at this stage. The widespread dissemination of prevention information that focuses on the risks and problems associated with abusing substances is the most effective way to slow the number of adolescents who move beyond this stage. In recent years, this area of prevention has been emphasized, raising adolescents' awareness of the potential dangers of general drug and alcohol use. More emphasis needs to be communicated on the specific dangers of using meth as the drug epidemic continues to escalate.

Stage 2: Regular Use

If the adolescent moves into a pattern of regular use, tolerance and a physical need or craving for the drug being abused can result. This happens most frequently with cigarettes, alcohol, and marijuana. However, adolescents who are pushing their experimental use of meth into regular use may easily miss the signals of an escalating dependence, which are often mistaken for anxiety, depression, and other psychological problems. In fact, these psychological problems are *caused* by the neurochemical imbalances created by meth abuse. This misattribution of symptoms gets in the way of people recognizing that their use has become a problem and seeking help.

A noticeable decline in functioning, a preoccupation with regular use (not necessarily *daily* with meth abusers), tolerance (the need to use more to continue to get the same effect), and the movement from using to experience pleasure to using to prevent negative feelings are indicators of a more significant problem. With meth abusers, the negative feelings often are experienced as depression, anxiety, paranoia, and other psychotic symptoms. Continued use relieves these symptoms in the same way that heroin relieves the flulike symptoms that signal opiate withdrawal.

The most effective approach for adolescents at this stage of abuse is a *selected prevention* approach. It should target people at risk for the particular illness—in this case, drug abuse. The idea is to provide new information about the illness that will motivate behavior change. This form of treatment is often offered as an early intervention. Evidence suggests that a relatively brief early intervention can be quite effective. Many of the adolescent treatments that have been developed to date are, in fact, early and brief interventions. (Some such treatments are described later in this chapter.) While these interventions have proven useful for young people who are abusing drugs such as marijuana and alcohol, little data is available on their effectiveness with meth users who have moved to the regular use stage. Many of the adolescents who are seeking assistance for their meth abuse prefer to enter a more intensive form of treatment. In general, however, it is more cost effective and easier to offer a brief intervention to a broader group of selected drug and alcohol abusers, especially when resources are limited. Future studies need to determine whether brief interventions are sufficient for adolescents who are regularly abusing meth.

Stage 3: Psychological and Physical Dependence

This is truly the stage at which the affected person can be said to be *addicted*. At this stage, there is a physiological or conditioned withdrawal. Keep in mind that the withdrawal symptoms of meth dependence often go unrecognized and are frequently misattributed. The depression, anxiety, and paranoia that accompany meth withdrawal are often not associated with the drug abuse. One of the hallmarks of this stage of dependence is that the drug use is associated with relief of or improvement in the withdrawal symptoms. Conversely, discontinuation of the drug use often results in recurrence of the symptoms. This is true of meth abuse, but it's difficult to use as a yardstick since the psychological symptoms are difficult for people to distinguish. At this stage of dependence, the abuser frequently progresses to abusing other illicit drugs. This is either an attempt to medicate the effects of the initially abused drug or a result of the increased availability of different drugs in his or her social environment. The latter is particularly true of adolescents who have gravitated to friends who are using and abusing a wide variety of drugs and alcohol.

Treatment for adolescents at this stage of drug abuse includes the range of treatment options that have been developed in the field to date. Primary treatment for adolescent substance abusers ranges from nonintensive outpatient treatment (characterized by regularly scheduled sessions for less than nine hours per week) to a group-home living situation (where participants live together in a treatment-oriented environment). There are other treatments that vary in intensity, content, and length of stay. The most common form of treatment for adolescents in the United States today is outpatient treatment (as opposed to residential or inpatient). Eight out of every ten adolescents in treatment in the United States are in some form of outpatient treatment. For this reason, this chapter focuses on what is known to date about the most effective forms of adolescent outpatient treatment.

Meth Task Force Recommendations

As noted in chapter 3, the Comprehensive Methamphetamine Control Act of 1996 authorized the formation of the Methamphetamine Interagency Task Force (MITF) in response to widespread meth use. One of this committee's tasks was to evaluate, design, and implement better treatment strategies specifically for meth abusers. These guidelines were published at www.ojp.usdoj.gov/nij/methintf/contents.html. They are listed below with comments regarding their application in the treatment of adolescents.

Treatment Must Be Guided by Research

> *Treatment of methamphetamine abusers should be guided by research findings. For circumstances in which there is no existing research evidence, treatment recommendations should be developed through a consensus process combining the opinions of professionals from research and clinical domains.*

Until very recently, the treatment of adolescents for drugs and alcohol, and for meth specifically, has fallen into the category of "circumstances in which there is no existing research evidence." In *Principles of Drug Addiction Treatment: A Research-Based Guide,* published by NIDA and available at www.nida.nih.gov/PODAT/PODATIndex.html, several promising practices for adolescents are mentioned.[2] Behavioral therapy has proven successful in research studies while using therapeutic activities such as fulfilling specific assignments, rehearsing desired behaviors, and praising plus rewarding achievement of goals. It has helped adolescents become drug free and remain that way after treatment ends. By including family members in therapy and rewarding drug abstinence as verified by urinalysis, adolescents have shown additional improvement in employment/school attendance, family relationships, and dealing with depression.

The NIDA booklet also describes two adolescent-specific therapies with research support. The first is Multidimensional Family Therapy (MDFT), a treatment in which adolescent drug use is viewed in terms of a network of influences (family, individual, peer, community). MDFT provides guidelines for both the adolescent and family members in the clinic, home, family court, school, or other community locations. The second is Multisystemic Therapy (MST), an intensive service that has proven effective in reducing the number of incarcerations and out-of-home placements of juveniles. In this paradigm, intense treatment is provided in the participant's natural environments (home, school, and neighborhood settings). The treatment addresses the factors associated with serious antisocial behavior in adolescents who abuse drugs. These factors include adolescent characteristics (e.g., attitudes toward drug use), family (poor discipline, family conflict, parental drug abuse), school (performance and attendance), and neighborhood (local criminal subculture).

More recently, SAMHSA funded a large-scale study through the Center for Substance Abuse Treatment (CSAT). It tested the effectiveness and cost-effectiveness of a variety of interventions targeted at reducing/eliminating marijuana use and associated problems in adolescents. The study, the Cannabis Youth Treatment (CYT) project, is a randomized field experiment.[3] The implementation of this large-scale study is an example of the next principle listed below.

Research Must Be Carefully Disseminated to Treatment Providers

> *While the United States has made great progress in drug treatment research, this research has not been consistently disseminated to and implemented by providers.*

In the specific instance of adolescent treatment, the CYT project was an effort to do just that while evaluating the intervention effectiveness. A combination of Motivational Enhancement Therapy, Cognitive Behavioral Therapy, Family Support Network (FSN), the Adolescent Community Reinforcement Approach (ACRA), and Multidimensional Family Therapy (MDFT) were used in the CYT. All of these treatments have some proven effectiveness. While data analysis is still ongoing from the first phase of this study and another phase is being conducted, CYT outcome data seem to indicate the following:

- Co-occurring problems were the norm and varied with substance use severity.
- Neither dosage nor type of treatment produced clear advantages.

- While more effective than many earlier outpatient treatments, more than two-thirds of the CYT adolescents were still having problems twelve months later.
- The interventions were successful and affordable in a wide range of settings.
- The initial treatment costs were quickly offset by reductions in other costs to society. For example, the most important reduced cost to society was fewer "days in a controlled environment," meaning both inpatient treatment and detention.
- Most of the change in problems and costs to society occurred during the active treatment phase (five to twelve weeks) and were sustained out to twelve months posttreatment.

While the CYT did not include meth abusers, the general findings indicate where to begin formulating studies and treatments for meth-using adolescents, such as

- adapting manual-guided therapies to improve treatment effectiveness
- using the CYT interventions to provide replicable models to help the field maintain quality while expanding treatment capacity
- providing an adequate dose of treatment for the majority of adolescents, (CYT interventions were not an adequate dose of treatment)
- providing a continuum of care and ongoing recovery management for adolescents

Meth Treatment Should Be Conducted by Knowledgeable Individuals

> *Treatment of methamphetamine abusers should be conducted by individuals who have accurate knowledge of the effects of methamphetamine abuse and how these effects impact treatment and recovery.*

If the users are adolescents, the treatment providers should have specific knowledge of adolescent treatment. In 2002, the Robert Wood Johnson Foundation provided a grant to Drug Strategies (a nonprofit research institute that promotes more effective approaches to the U.S. drug problem) to identify the key elements in effective adolescent treatment programs and to observe how they are actually implemented in 144 recommended programs across the United States. One of the exemplary adolescent programs was developed by the Matrix Institute, an organization that has a long history of working with meth abusers in outpatient settings. Young meth addicts who participated in the Matrix adolescent program (which is being developed into a manual that will be published in 2005) are described in a recent article comparing them to program participants using substances other than meth. The article concludes that prior to treatment, the meth-using adolescents tended to be more psychologically impaired then their non-meth-using counterparts. They had histories of more exposure to physical and sexual abuse and more serious legal and school problems. Because of this, the meth-abusing adolescents may well need special treatment programming.[4]

Treatment Needs to Be Meth-Specific

> *Treatment strategies should incorporate and reflect the unique problems facing methamphetamine abusers during their recovery, including the mental health issues often produced by methamphetamine abuse.*

The Drug Strategies publication *Treating Teens: A Guide to Adolescent Drug Programs* outlines nine key elements that contribute to effective treatment. These elements were drawn from research and clinical practice as studied and reported by their distinguished advisory panel of nationally recognized experts. The key elements are

- providing thorough assessment and treatment matching
- using comprehensive, integrated treatment approaches
- encouraging family involvement in treatment
- providing developmentally appropriate programming
- fostering relationships that engage and retain teens in treatment
- hiring qualified staff
- designing programs that address gender and cultural differences
- developing activities that will provide continuing care
- conducting treatment outcomes[5]

In addition to these adolescent-specific issues, programs treating meth-abusing teens also need to address the increased psychosocial dysfunctionality that is apparent in this population (auditory hallucinations, depression, suicidality, school problems, legal dilemmas, and so on).

Treatment Should Be Comprehensive

> *To ensure maximum effectiveness and efficiency of treatment, methamphetamine abusers must have access to a full continuum of care. In addition, treatment should include case management and links to primary care and mental health services, as appropriate. Treatment should also be culturally appropriate and encourage the participation of family members and others close to the abuser.*

In addition to the CYT project mentioned earlier, CSAT is undertaking a large-scale project evaluating ten exemplary adolescent treatment programs in the United States. The Adolescent Treatment Models (ATM) program is designed to evaluate, document, and disseminate effective adolescent substance abuse treatment models. The ten programs participating in this study provide comprehensive care in a variety of settings: three outpatient programs; one family-oriented treatment program (MDFT, mentioned earlier); three residential treatment programs; and three modified therapeutic community treatment models. Upon completion, the participating programs will receive assistance from CSAT in developing manuals outlining their programs and in disseminating those materials.[6]

Appropriate Treatment Should Be Provided in the Criminal Justice System

> *Scientific studies demonstrate that appropriately treating incarcerated addicts reduces their later drug abuse by between 50 and 70 percent and their later criminality and resulting re-arrests by between 50 and 60 percent.*

Almost half the adolescents abusing meth who enter publicly funded substance abuse treatment programs are involved with the juvenile justice system. Appropriate treatment involves more than the problems specific to substance abuse. Those adolescents also need help for family relationship problems, scholastic issues, and learning new prosocial behaviors. In many states, juvenile justice systems are anchored by juvenile drug courts. Drug courts recommend and oversee treatment referrals to a youth authority (state prison for adolescents), juvenile camps, residential community treatment settings, and, the least restrictive option, release with community supervision.

Treatment for Parents Is a Form of Prevention for Children

> *Research has shown that parental influence is a major factor in children's drug abuse patterns. Treatment programs for parents enhance protective factors among young children by removing them from a drug-taking environment and by teaching parents skills for avoiding drug abuse.*

For adolescents, family involvement is a strong factor in ensuring both treatment retention and success. A recent study of adolescents who stopped using drugs without formal treatment showed that the three most important factors supporting their efforts were parental involvement, new friends, and motivation. Prevention programs that focus on teaching parents behavioral strategies and methods for using positive reinforcement have been shown to be very effective in deterring adolescents from drug and alcohol abuse.

Treatment Should Address the Needs of At-Risk Groups

> *Methamphetamine has impacted a number of specific population groups to a disproportionate degree according to anecdotal reports; therefore, treatment for methamphetamine abusers should consider the needs of severely impacted groups.*

Female adolescent drug users are particularly impacted by meth use. At least one study shows that female adolescents abusing meth tend to enter treatment identifying meth as a primary problem more frequently than males. Once in treatment, females tend to focus on relationship issues. These issues were not historically addressed in a system that was initially designed for adult males. Another highly affected group of adolescent drug users are those who use experimentally and relatively infrequently. This large group comprises the "at-risk" youth who need to be educated about meth and motivated to change their risky behavior. Motivational enhancement techniques have been proven effective and are an important element in the highly successful brief interventions used to deter adolescent drug use. The hallmark of this style is a nonconfrontational, collegial approach to developing an empathic relationship. It provides important personalized information to the adolescent in a way that does not cause defensiveness or further rebellion.

Treatment in Rural Areas Poses Particular Problems

> *In rural areas, access to and availability of health care in general and substance abuse treatment in particular are problematic. For example, geographical distances between providers and those in need of services, the lack of continuing training for providers, and the need for residential treatment all contribute to the problem.*

Few good answers have been found to date for this problem of servicing adolescents who live in remote and rural areas. CSAT's ATM study (described earlier) includes several programs that employ a "step-down" approach to treatment. This may offer some hope for adolescents who are fortunate enough to receive residential treatment and then have to face the very real problems encountered upon reentry into their families and communities. The newly developing field of telemedicine can be useful in rural areas. With modern telecommunication technology, people who otherwise would be unable to access professional help can now receive it.

Clearly, there are many unanswered and unformed questions as to how we can most effectively and efficiently treat the increasing number of adolescent meth abusers. The number of adolescent meth users continues to rise, and the multitude of problems that accompany the trend increases. This problem will not go away on its own. The efforts of the U.S. government and of treatment programs to find solutions to the myriad issues involved are critical to the success of this important work.

CHAPTER SIX

CHILDREN AND METH

by Patricia Marinelli-Casey and Nena Messina

Meth now ranks as the most widely abused illicit drug in much of the western United States, and its use is increasing in other parts of the nation.[1] According to the World Health Organization, more than thirty-five million people worldwide regularly use meth. The effects and consequences of meth dependence have been well documented and publicized. However, less attention has been given to the countless number of children who have been directly affected by the epidemic. This is of particular concern since more and more women of childbearing age have selected meth as their drug of choice.[2] Infants born to meth-using mothers generally have a higher risk for low birth weight and developmental and behavioral problems. In addition, the reported number of children present at seized meth labs across the United States has increased dramatically, from 950 in 1999 to more than 3,000 in 2002.[3] Increased meth use and home-based production has resulted in an escalation of reported serious child abuse and neglect. Children living in meth labs are at extremely high risk for poisoning, homicide, and accidental deaths and burns due to methamphetamine lab fires and explosions.

Maternal Meth Use Consequences

Research on the general development of children exposed to drugs, both pre- and postnatally, is sparse, particularly with regard to meth exposure. Much of the literature on drug-exposed children focuses on the effects of prenatal cocaine or opiate exposure.[4] However, some studies have assessed the effects of meth-exposed infants compared with non-meth-exposed infants in utero. Similar to cocaine exposure, prenatal exposure to meth is associated with premature delivery, complications during pregnancy, altered neonatal behavioral patterns (e.g., abnormal reflexes and extreme irritability), low birth weight, and smaller head circumference.[5] Oro and Dixon further reported that neonates exposed to meth demonstrated neurological and physiological abnormalities such as disruptive sleep patterns, poor feeding, and tremors.[6] It is not clear whether these early symptoms of meth exposure resolve over time or lead to long-term developmental problems.

Preliminary data from the Prenatal Methamphetamine Project found that prenatal exposure to meth was associated with small but significant decrements in cognitive, language, and behavioral functioning in children ages three to six years old.[7] Pilot data provide support for a more complete and definitive examination of how pre- and postnatal meth exposure affect child development. However, interpretation of the research on drug-exposed children is difficult because of poor maternal health, inadequate nutrition, and overall family dysfunction.[8]

A Swedish retrospective study of children followed meth-exposed children to the age of fourteen. As early as age four, these children exhibited aggressive behaviors associated with longer periods of exposure to meth in utero. Compared with non-meth-exposed children, the exposed children were held back in school more often due to delays in language and math skills.[9]

Meth Labs

Scope of the Problem

Drug Enforcement Administration (DEA) meth lab seizures in the United States rose from 549 in 1990 to 2,155 in 1999.[10] With widely available meth recipes on the Internet and elsewhere, a virtual cottage industry of home-based meth labs has emerged. Meth is easily manufactured with inexpensive over-the-counter ingredients, although recent legislation has restricted large-quantity purchases of meth precursors.

There are two primary methods of meth production: P-2-P (phenyl-2-propanone) and ephedrine reduction. The processes received their names from the precursor chemicals used in the production of the drug. Since the possession or purchase of P-2-P is now illegal in the United States, this method is used primarily by large drug cartels in Mexico. Ephedrine reduction has become the primary method of production in the United States, where manufacturers known as "cooks" chemically extract ephedrine or pseudoephedrine from over-the-counter cold medicines. Once the ephedrine has been extracted, it is combined with various reaction agents to produce meth.

There are two methods commonly used to produce meth: red phosphorous (Red P) and Nazi (dry cook). The red phosphorous method involves combining ephedrine or pseudoephedrine with red phosphorous and hydriodic acid. Red phosphorous is usually extracted from match tips, computer chips, flares, and fireworks. The Nazi method uses ephedrine or pseudoephedrine, sodium or lithium, and anhydrous ammonia. Lithium strips are usually extracted from batteries. Other ingredients commonly used in meth production include items such as denatured alcohol, ether, salt, drain cleaner, paint thinner, lye, Freon, and camping fuel. The use of a particular method of production varies by geographic region and appears to be dependent upon the availability of chemicals necessary for the manufacturing process.

All of the substances mentioned above are highly toxic, corrosive, and/or flammable. In fact, many labs are found because of fire or explosion. In several states, meth production is legally categorized as an "inherently dangerous felony" because of these known dangers. In addition, many of the chemicals used in meth production are restricted by Occupational Safety and Health Administration (OSHA) regulations, which require that hazardous materials teams clean up meth lab sites. As noted earlier, five to seven pounds of toxic waste are generated for each pound of meth manufactured.[11] This waste is commonly dumped in backyards, Dumpsters, storm drains, parks, or along roadsides and farm fields, where it is a source of long-lasting and toxic pollution. Chemical contamination also occurs indoors where the meth is made, with measurable contamination remaining years after labs are shut down.

Dangers of Labs and Special Risks to Children

One of the most pernicious and little-examined consequences of the meth abuse/production epidemic is the endangerment of children. According to both researchers and law enforcement reports, increased use of meth across the United States has resulted in a dramatic escalation in the severity of child abuse crimes and an increase in child abuse homicides.[12] Children are more likely to be exposed to home-based meth labs than larger clandestine drug labs.[13] Besides being exposed to meth and the toxic precursor chemicals used in its production, these children are often the victims of their parents' drug-focused lifestyles, which are often characterized by neglect, physical or sexual abuse, domestic violence, and other criminal activities.[14] In addition, children of drug-dependent parents are at high risk to continue intergenerational patterns of drug abuse, criminal behaviors, and neglectful parenting.[15]

Health Risks of Meth Lab Exposure

The immediate dangers to children posed by home-based meth labs extend beyond the violence, neglect, and abuse associated with drug-abusing and drug-selling activities. Children who live in meth labs are also exposed to the toxic chemicals, waste, and filth associated with meth production, as well as to the highly psychoactive stimulant itself. Accidental ingestion can cause psychosis, seizures, and death.[16] Consequences of exposure to the toxic precursor chemicals can include poisoning, burns, and lung irritation; damage to the liver, kidneys, heart, brain, and immune system; cancers such as lymphoma and leukemia; bone marrow suppression resulting in anemia and increased risk of infections; and developmental and growth problems.[17]

The conditions of the typical meth home environment can further increase a child's risk of infection and illness. Lack of cleanliness is customary, providing an atmosphere for pests and bacteria to thrive. Domestic animals contribute to the filth, particularly dogs, which are often used to protect the drug lab from intruders. Commonly, animal feces, ticks, fleas, garbage, rotten food, cockroaches, and discarded drug paraphernalia are present in the child's living areas.[18] Personal hygiene is poor and lack of parental supervision contributes to a high percentage of children ingesting spoiled, rotten, or chemically contaminated food, as meth solutions are often stored in real food containers.[19]

Table 7 outlines factors that increase health risks for children as compared to adults in the same residence.

Effects of Parental Neglect and Abuse

Neglected and abused children are at risk of social, emotional, developmental, and behavioral problems during childhood and adolescence, as well as cognitive damage, psychological damage, and permanent brain damage or physical impairments.[20] The most severe consequence of neglect and abuse is death.[21]

Neglect is often viewed as separate from physical abuse.[22] In the past, neglect was not considered to be as serious as abuse.[23] However, recent research has shown that neglect in the early stages of life may lead to severe, chronic,

TABLE 7

Additional Health Risks to Children, Compared to Adults[24]

GROWING AND DEVELOPING ORGANISMS:
Children's body size, higher rate of growth and development, and faster metabolism and breathing rate mean they are more likely to absorb higher doses of the chemicals and drugs than adults. The developing brain and other organ systems are more susceptible to damage at specific maturational levels. Children may not be able to process and eliminate the chemicals as well as adults and are therefore also at risk of neurological and developmental problems.
SPECIFIC BEHAVIORS:
Methamphetamine and many of the chemicals involved in its manufacture are absorbed through the skin. Because young children have more contact than adults with their physical environment—on the floor, soil, and other surfaces, like beds, countertops, and low tables—they are likely to be exposed to more of the drug and contaminants in their homes. Young children are also much more likely to put their hands or chemically contaminated objects in their mouths and to be accidentally poisoned by ingesting the drug, an intermediate meth solution, or chemicals that can be fatal or life threatening.
DIFFERENTIAL LIFE SPAN:
Children have a much longer life span than adults, during which chemical exposure can lead to acute or chronic effects or cancers.
VULNERABILITY:
Children are more likely to be neglected, abused, or molested while living in homes of meth "cookers." Such environments are often chaotic and drug focused, and the lifestyle associated with severe meth dependency tends to be one of disorganization, irritability, instability, and violence.
INEXPERIENCE:
Young children are less likely to be able to escape from or survive a lab-related fire or explosion due to their inexperience in emergencies; they are also less likely to be rescued due to their parents' inability to think clearly when under the influence of meth.

and irreversible damage.[25] Consistent with attachment theory,[26] which describes the effects of early parent-child connections, parental neglect occurring early in life is particularly detrimental to subsequent development and later attachment to others. For example, relative to physical abuse, neglect is more often associated with developmental delays (i.e., in regard to the normal progression of developmental milestones), with severe cognitive and academic deficits, and with social withdrawal throughout childhood and early adolescence.[27] Physical consequences of neglect arise because of lack of nutrition or emotional stimulation. This can alter the release of important growth-regulating hormones and influence the physical development of the body, including the brain.[28] The impact of child neglect can vary depending on the child and on the remedial and enrichment experiences provided after the neglect occurs.[29]

Abused children are typically neglected as well; however, the reverse is not necessarily as common. Children who survive both abuse and neglect are at risk of a multitude of emotional and behavioral problems. Abused and neglected children are often angry, antisocial, hyperactive, physically aggressive, and even violent.[30] In addition, they often perform poorly in school and engage in delinquent behavior.[31] For some, the consequences include low self-esteem, depression, hopelessness, self-mutilation, and suicide attempts.[32] Studies have also linked childhood abuse and neglect to compulsiveness, panic attacks, personality disorders, dissociation, and dangerous play.[33] Cumulatively, the increased likelihood for aggression and disciplinary problems places these children at a much greater risk for criminal involvement later in life.[34]

The effects of abuse and neglect range in severity, often depending on the age of exposure (or the developmental period), the chronicity of maltreatment, and/or the gender of the child. For example, severe maltreatment occurring in the early childhood years, when the child and the brain are most rapidly developing, is particularly detrimental to successful adaptation.[35] Other research suggests that chronicity, rather than type or severity, of maltreatment is the strongest predictor of negative outcomes for children.[36] Finally, little attention has been paid to how boys and girls may differ in their response and adaptation to experiences of abuse and neglect. Wolfe and McGee found a significant interaction between gender and the timing and the nature of childhood maltreatment on subsequent adolescent adjustment.[37] For boys, poor adolescent adjustment was related to physical and psychological abuse, neglect, and witnessing spousal abuse during early childhood. For girls, poor adolescent adjustment was related to neglect or psychological abuse during midchildhood. Childhood maltreatment poses additional risks for girls, as physical and sexual abuse during childhood have consistently been linked to a cycle of later victimization by domestic partners.[38] Sexual abuse has also been found to be related to post-traumatic stress disorder (PTSD) and sexual promiscuity in adolescent girls.[39] Moreover, early sexual abuse is a stronger predictor of later criminal activity for women than for men.[40]

Exposure to Domestic Violence

It is estimated that between three and ten million children in the United States witness acts of domestic violence every year,[41] and the correlations between domestic violence, substance abuse, and child abuse are well documented.[42] Recent evidence identifies a strong link between domestic violence and meth use specifically. For example, police in Contra Costa County, California, report that meth use is involved in almost 90 percent of the domestic dispute cases investigated by that agency.[43] Current research suggests how exposure to domestic violence may affect a child's adjustment and adaptation. The literature cites short- and long-term effects, including social withdrawal (or detachment) and lack of bonding with parents (either the perpetrator or the victim) in early childhood and chronic anxiety, eating disorders, sleeping disorders, depression, aggression, self-destructive behavior, PTSD, and school problems in later years.[44] In addition, witnessing violence in childhood is associated with, for boys, perpetrating violence in adulthood and, for girls, continued victimization.[45] However, given the strong connection between domestic violence and parental substance abuse, the effects of witnessing domestic violence during childhood are multidimensional and complex.

Help for the Children: Drug Endangered Children Initiative

In 1997, the California Governor's Office of Criminal Justice Planning funded a three-year pilot called the Drug Endangered Children (DEC) project. Seven county-based multidisciplinary response teams (DEC teams) were developed and trained to protect children found living in drug manufacturing, selling, and abusing homes. The pilot teams (in Los Angeles, San Diego, San Bernardino, Riverside, Butte, Orange, and Shasta Counties) included narcotics officers, child protective services (CPS) personnel, medical professionals, and prosecutors.

Providing twenty-four-hour on-scene response at meth lab seizures, the teams worked to reduce child trauma and provide timely medical evaluations of children, as well as to ensure that prosecutors filed felony child endangerment charges. In addition, a DEC Resource Center was developed and provided ongoing training, educational materials, and medical protocols to the DEC teams.

The California pilot counties have served nearly four thousand children, many of whom have needed special counseling and developmental services. Preliminary data indicates that 38 percent of the children removed from home-based meth labs tested positive for meth and exhibited a higher-than-expected incidence of respiratory, dermatological, and dental problems.[46] Reports also show that young children were exposed to meth primarily through second-hand smoke, accidental ingestion, skin absorption through direct contact, and food and beverage contamination. According to a preliminary analysis of ninety-five DEC cases in San Bernardino County, 43 percent of children found in meth labs had abnormal initial medical exam results following the lab seizure, and 42 percent (N=50) had developmental delays or cautions. In San Diego County, 472 children were found in 176 homes during meth lab seizures and were removed by child welfare officials during a two-year period (1997–1999). More than one-third of these children tested positive for illicit drugs. Of these children, 386 had dependency petitions filed and sustained in juvenile court.[47]

As of 2004, DEC response teams operate fifteen of California's fifty-eight counties, which has resulted in the formation of the California DEC Alliance, an ad hoc group of California DEC practitioners promoting the expansion of DEC programs. In addition, DEC training originating from the California DEC Resource Center has occurred in eighteen states, and DEC programs currently operate formally in California, Washington, Oregon, Idaho, Arizona, Utah, Colorado, Oklahoma, Missouri, and Illinois. Since the 1997 DEC pilot study, the DEC response teams have operated as a collection of local initiatives.

The DEC program has continued to grow through the dedication and determination of concerned individuals, despite inadequate funding. Communities throughout the United States have sought training to meet the needs of children affected by the methamphetamine epidemic. A national DEC training coordinator is now available to disseminate information, provide training, and assist counties in developing DEC response teams. The national DEC training coordinator is located in the United States Attorney's Office, Department of Justice, in San Diego, California. For more information, write to National DEC Training Coordinator, 880 Front Street, Room 6293, San Diego, CA 92101-8893, or call (619) 557-7736.

■ ■ ■

NOTES

Chapter 1: Methamphetamine 101: The Basics

1. M. S. Gold and N. S. Miller, "Cocaine (and Crack): Neurobiology," in *Substance Abuse: A Comprehensive Textbook,* ed. J. H. Lowinson, P. Ruiz, R. B. Millman, and J. G. Langrod (Baltimore, MD: Williams & Wilkins, 1977).

2. Ibid.

3. Gold and Miller, "Cocaine (and Crack)"; B. Sowder and G. Beschner, eds., "Methamphetamine: An Illicit Drug with High Abuse Potential, unpublished report from NIDA contract no. 271-9-002" (Rockville, MD: T. Head and Company, Inc., 1993).

Chapter 2: Clinical Challenges in Treating Meth Abusers

1. R. A. Rawson et al., "Neurobehavioral Treatment for Cocaine Dependency," *Journal of Psychoactive Drugs* 22 (1990): 159–71.

2. Substance Abuse and Mental Health Services Administration (SAMHSA), *Drug Abuse Warning Network,* http://dawninfo.samhsa.gov.

3. R. A. Rawson et al., "A Multisite Comparison of Psychosocial Approaches for the Treatment of Methamphetamine Dependence," *Addiction* 99 (2004): 708–17.

4. D. S. Bell, "The Experimental Reproduction of Amphetamine Psychosis," *Archives of General Psychiatry* 29 (1973): 35–40; J. D. Griffith et al., "Dextroamphetamine: Evaluation of Psychomimetic Properties in Man," *Archives of General Psychiatry* 26 (1972): 97–100; W. Hall et al., "Psychological Morbidity and Route of Administration among Amphetamine Users in Sydney, Australia," *Addiction* 91 (1996): 81–87.

5. D. S. Bell, "Comparison of Amphetamine Psychosis and Schizophrenia," *British Journal of Psychiatry* 111 (1965): 701–7; S. H. Snyder, "Amphetamine Psychosis: A 'Model' Schizophrenia Medicated by Cathecholamines," *American Journal of Psychiatry* 130 (1973): 61–67.

6. M. Sato et al., "Acute Exacerbation of Paranoid Psychotic State after Long-Term Abstinence in Patients with Previous Methamphetamine Psychosis," *Biological Psychiatry* 18, no. 4 (1983): 429–40.

7. D. A. Regier et al., "Comorbidity of Mental Disorders with Alcohol and Other Drug Abuse: Results for the Epidemiologic Catchment Area (ECA) Study," *Journal of the American Medical Association* 264 (1990): 2511–18.

8. B. J. Rounsaville et al., "Heterogeneity of Psychiatric Diagnosis in Treated Opiate Addicts," *Archives of General Psychiatry* 390 (1982): 161–68.

9. K. T. Muesser et al., "Prevalence of Substance Abuse in Schizophrenia, Demographic and Clinical Correlates," *Schizophrenia Bulletin* 6 (1990): 10–41; J. A. Selzer and J. A. Lieberman, "Schizophrenia and Substance Abuse," *Psychiatric Clinics of North America* 16 (1993): 401–12.

10. R. K. Brooner et al., "Psychiatric and Substance Abuse Comorbidity among Treatment-Seeking Opioid Abusers," *Archives of General Psychiatry* 54 (1997): 71–80.

11. For more information about MCTG and the current and upcoming trials within this multisite research group, visit www.clinicaltrials.gov or www.uclaisap.org, or contact the UCLA ISAP Research Group at (888) 333-1764. To contact NIDA, write to Division of Treatment Research and Development, National Institute on Drug Abuse, National Institutes of Health, 6001 Executive Boulevard, Room 4133, Bethesda, MD 20892, or call (301) 443-1124.

Chapter 4: Assessment: Getting It Right

1. R. A. Rawson, P. Marinelli-Casey, and A. Huber, "A Multisite Evaluation of Treatment of Methamphetamine Dependence in Adults," in *Conducting Multiple Site Evaluations in Real-World Settings,* ed. J. M. Herrell and R. B. Straw (San Francisco, CA: Jossey-Bass, 2002), 73–87; R. A. Rawson, P. Marinelli-Casey, and A. Huber, "Treating Methamphetamine Dependence in Adults," in *Planning and Managing Multi-site Trials,* ed. R. Straw and J. Herrell (San Francisco, CA: Jossey-Bass, 2002), 93.

2. Center for Substance Abuse Treatment, "Proceedings of the National Consensus Meeting on the Use, Abuse, and Sequelae of Abuse of Methamphetamine with Implications for Prevention, Treatment, and Research," DHHS pub. no. (SMA) 96-8013 (Rockville, MD: CSAT, Substance Abuse and Mental Health Services Administration, Department of Health and Human Services, 1997).

3. American Psychiatric Association, *Diagnostic and Statistical Manual of Mental Disorders,* 4th ed., text revision (Washington, DC: American Psychiatric Association, 2000).

4. A. T. McLellan, H. Kushner, and D. Metzger, "The Fifth Edition of the Addiction Severity Index," *Substance Abuse Treatment* 9 (1992): 199–213.

5. Ibid.

6. A. M. Washton, N. S. Stone, and E. C. Hendrickson, "Cocaine Abuse," in *Assessment of Addictive Behaviors,* ed. D. M. Donovan and G. A. Marlatt (New York: Guilford Press, 1988), 364–89.

7. M. Freire-Garabal et al., "Effects of Amphetamine on Development of Oral Candidiasis in Rats," *Clinical and Diagnostic Laboratory Immunology* 6 (1999): 530–33; P. J. Redfearn, N. Agrawal, and L. H. Mair, "An Association between the Regular Use of 3,4 Methylenedioxy-Methamphetamine (Ecstasy) and Excessive Wear of the Teeth," *Addiction* 92 (1998): 745–48; G. W. Ashcroft, D. Eccleston, and

J. L. Waddell, "Recognition of Amphetamine Addicts," *British Medical Journal* 1 (1965): 57; S. J. See and E. K. Tan, "Severe Amphetamine-Induced Bruxism: Treatment with Botulinum Toxin," *Acta Neurologica Scandinavica* 107 (2003): 161–63.

8. P. H. Connell, *Amphetamine Psychosis* (London: Chapmann and Hall, 1958); D. Fujii, "Risk Factors for Treatment-Resistant Methamphetamine Psychosis," *Journal of Neuropsychiatry and Clinical Neurosciences* 14 (2002): 239–40; A. Iwanami et al., "Patients with Methamphetamine Psychosis Admitted to a Psychiatric Hospital in Japan: A Preliminary Report," *Acta Psychiatric Scandinavica* 89 (1994): 428–32.

9. S. L. Sate, W. M. Southwick, and F. H. Gain, "Clinical Features of Cocaine-Induced Paranoia," *American Journal of Psychiatry* 148 (1991): 495–98.

10. F. Gain, M. Khalsa, and E. Ellinwood, "Stimulants and Related Drugs," in *Synopsis of Treatments of Psychiatric Disorders,* ed. G. O. Gabbard and S. D. Atkinson (Washington, DC: American Psychiatric Press, 1996), 313–28; Y. Sekine et al., "Methamphetamine-Related Psychiatric Symptoms and Reduced Brain Dopamine Transporters Studied with PET," *American Journal of Psychiatry* 158 (2001): 1206–14.

11. A. Buffenstein, J. Heaster, and P. Ko, "Chronic Psychotic Illness from Methamphetamine," *American Journal of Psychiatry* 156 (1999): 662.

12. Iwanami et al., "Patients with Methamphetamine Psychosis," 428–32.

13. Fujii, "Risk Factors," 239–40.

14. S. L. Simon et al., "Cognitive Impairment in Individuals Currently Using Methamphetamine," *American Journal on Addictions* 9 (2000): 222–31.

15. G. R. King and E. H. Ellinwood Jr., "Amphetamines and Other Stimulants," in *Substance Abuse: A Comprehensive Textbook,* ed. J. H. Lowinson, P. Ruiz, R. B. Millman, and J. G. Langrod (Baltimore, MD: Williams & Wilkins, 1992), 247–70.

16. E. London et al., "Regional Cerebral Dysfunction Associated with Mood Disturbances in Abstinent Methamphetamine Abusers," *Archives of General Psychiatry* 61 (2004): 73–84.

17. R. A. Rawson, R. G. Gonzales, and P. Brethen, "Methamphetamine: Current Research Findings and Clinical Challenges," *Journal of Substance Abuse Treatment* 23 (2002): 145–50.

Chapter 5: Adolescents and Meth

1. N. A. Kaczynski and C. S. Martin, "Diagnostic Orphans: Adolescents with Clinical Alcohol Symptomatology Who Do Not Quality for *DSM-IV* Abuse or Dependence Diagnosis" (paper presented at the annual meeting of the Research Society on Alcoholism, Steamboat Springs, CO, June 1995); C. S. Martin et al., "Polydrug Use in Adolescent Drinkers with and without *DSM-IV* Alcohol Abuse and Dependence," *Alcoholism: Clinical and Experimental Research* 20 (1996): 1099–1108; K. C. Winters, W. W. Latimer, and R. D. Stinchfield, "*DSM-IV* Criteria for Adolescent

Alcohol and Cannabis Use Disorders," *Journal of Studies on Alcohol* 60 (1999): 337–334.

2. National Institute on Drug Abuse, *Principles of Drug Addiction Treatment: A Research-Based Guide,* NIH publication no. 00-4180 (Bethesda, MD: National Institute on Drug Abuse, 1999).

3. M. Dennis et al., *Main Findings of the Cannabis Youth Treatment (CYT) Randomized Field Experiment, Proceedings of the American Psychiatric Association Annual Conference* (Philadelphia: U.S. Department of Health and Human Services, 2002).

4. R. A. Rawson et al., "Methamphetamine Use among Treatment-Seeking Adolescents in Southern California: Participant Characteristics and Treatment Response" (paper submitted).

5. Drug Strategies, *Treating Teens: A Guide to Adolescent Drug Programs* (Washington, DC: Robert Wood Johnson, 2003).

6. S. J. Stevens and A. R. Morral, eds., *Adolescent Substance Abuse Treatment in the United States* (New York: Hayworth, 2003).

Chapter 6: Children and Meth

1. Office of National Drug Control Policies, *Trends in Drug Abuse* (Rockville, MD: Drug Policy Information Clearinghouse, 2003); R. A. Rawson, M. D. Anglin, and W. Ling, "Will the Methamphetamine Problem Go Away?" *Journal of Addictive Diseases* 21 (2002): 5–19.

2. M. Hohman, R. Oliver, and W. Wright, "Methamphetamine Abuse, Manufacture, and the Child Welfare Response," *Social Work* (in press).

3. El Paso Intelligence Center National Clandestine Laboratory Seizure System, statistics, www.usdoj.gov/dea.

4. R. P. Barth and B. Needell, "Outcomes for Drug-Exposed Children Four Years Post-Adoption," *Children and Youth Services Review* 18, nos. 1 and 2 (1996): 37–56; B. Lester et al., "The Maternal Lifestyle Study: Effects of Substance Exposure during Pregnancy on Neurodevelopmental Outcome in 1-month-old Infants," *Pediatrics* 110, no. 6 (2002): 1182–92; B. Lester et al., "The Maternal Lifestyle Study: Effects of Prenatal Cocaine and/or Opiate Exposure on Auditory Brain Response at One Month," *Journal of Pediatrics* 142, no. 3 (2003): 279–85.

5. M. Eriksson, G. Larsson, and R. Zetterstrom, "Amphetamine Addiction and Pregnancy," *Acta Obstetricia et Gynecologoca Scandinavica* 60 (1981): 253; Hohman, Oliver, and Wright, "Methamphetamine Abuse"; A. S. Oro and S. D. Dixon, "Perinatal Cocaine and Methamphetamine Exposure: Maternal and Neonatal Correlates," *Journal of Pediatrics* 111 (1987): 57–58; L. Smith et al., "Effects of Prenatal Methamphetamine Exposure on Fetal Growth and Drug Withdrawal Symptoms in Infants Born at Term," *Journal of Developmental and Behavioral Pediatrics* 24 (2003): 17–23.

6. Oro and Dixon, "Perinatal Cocaine and Methamphetamine Exposure," 57–58.

7. R. Rawson, "A Pilot Study on the Impact of Prenatal Methamphetamine Exposure on the Cognitive, Language, and Behavioral Development of Pre-school Aged Children," presented at the Regional Methamphetamine Conference: Knowledge, Strategies, and Treatment for a Growing Community Problem, Kapolei, HI, December 1999.

8. R. P. Barth, "Research Outcomes of Prenatal Substance Exposure and the Need to Review Policies and Procedures Regarding Child Abuse Reporting," *Child Welfare* 80, no. 2 (2001): 275–96; Barth and Needell, "Outcomes for Drug-Exposed Children Four Years Post-Adoption"; D. Brooks and R. P. Barth, "Characteristics and Outcomes of Drug-Exposed and Non Drug-Exposed Children in Kinship and Non-relative Foster Care," *Children and Youth Services Review* 20, no. 6 (1998): 475–501; Rawson, "A Pilot Study on the Impact"; N. K. Young, "Effects of Alcohol and Other Drugs on Children," *Journal of Psychoactive Drugs* 29, no. 1 (1997): 23–42.

9. L. Cernerud et al., "Amphetamine Addiction during Pregnancy: 14-Year Follow-Up of Growth and School Performance," *Acta Paediatrica* 85 (1996): 204–8.

10. Drug Enforcement Agency, statistics, www.usdoj.gov/dea (2002).

11. Governor's Office of Criminal Justice Planning Guidebook, *Linking Drugs with Child Endangerment* (Sacramento, CA: 1999).

12. National Center on Addiction and Substance Abuse at Columbia University, *No Safe Haven: Children of Substance-Abusing Parents* (New York: National Center on Addiction and Substance Abuse, 1999); M. Petit and P. Curtis, *Child Abuse and Neglect: A Look at the States* (Washington, DC: Child Welfare League of America, 1997).

13. Department of Justice Information Bulletin, *Children at Risk,* pub. no. 2002-L0424-001, 2002.

14. R. L. Hampton, V. Senatore, and T. P. Gullota, *Substance Abuse, Family Violence, and Child Welfare: Bridging Perspectives* (Thousand Oaks, CA: Sage Publications, 1998); A. Shillington, M. Hohman, and L. Jones, "Women in Substance Use Treatment: Are Those Involved in the Child Welfare System Different?" *Journal of Social Work Practice in the Addictions* 1, no. 4 (2001): 25–46; A. Rosas, "Child Sexual Abuse," in *Child Abuse and Neglect: Guidelines for the Identification, Assessment, and Case Management,* ed. M. Durfee and M. Peterson (Vocano, CA: Volcano Press, 2003); A. Rosas, "Sexually Transmitted Diseases," in *Child Abuse and Neglect: Guidlines for the Identification, Assessment, and Case Management,* ed. M. Durfee and M. Peterson (Vocano, CA: Volcano Press, 2003).

15. M. Dunn et al., "Origins and Consequences of Child Neglect in Substance Abuse Families," *Clinical Psychology Review* 22 (2002): 1063–90; S. Greene, C. Haney, and A. Hurtado, "Cycles of Pain: Risk Factors in the Lives of Incarcerated Mothers and Their Children," *The Prison Journal* 80, no. 1 (2000): 3–23; M. J. Sheridan, "Proposed Intergenerational Model of Substance Abuse, Family Functioning, and Abuse/Neglect," *Child Abuse and Neglect* 19, no. 5 (1995): 519–30.

16. National Institute on Drug Abuse, Research Report Series, *Methamphetamine Abuse and Addiction,* NIH publication no. 02-4210 (Bethesda, MD: National Institute on Drug Abuse, 2002); J. A. Perez, E. L. Assure, and S. Strategies, "Methamphetamine-Related Stroke: Four Cases," *Journal of Emergency Medicine* 17, no. 3 (1999): 469–71.

17. Drug Endangered Children (DEC), *Drug Endangered Children Health and Safety Manual,* 2000 (previously available from the Drug Endangered Children Resource Center, 14622 Victory Blvd., Van Nuys, CA 91411); G. D. Irvine and L. Chin, "The Environmental Impact and Adverse Health Effects of the Clandestine Manufacture of Methamphetamine," *Substance Use and Misuse* 32, nos. 12 and 13 (1997): 1811–12; National Institute on Drug Abuse, *Methamphetamine Abuse and Addiction.*

18. T. Manning, "Drug Labs and Endangered Children," in *FBI Law Enforcement Bulletin* (1999), 10–14; E. Mendoza, personal communication, May 15, 2003.

19. Department of Justice Information Bulletin, *Children at Risk,* pub. no. 2002-L0424-001, 2002; Manning, "Drug Labs," 10–14.

20. Dunn et al., "Origins and Consequences of Child Neglect," 1063–90; K. Hildyard and D. Wolfe, "Child Neglect: Developmental Issues and Outcomes," *Child Abuse and Neglect* 26 (2002): 679–95.

21. T. O. Ireland, "Child Maltreatment," in *Encyclopedia of Crime and Punishment,* vol. 1, ed. D. Levinson (Great Barrington, MA: Berkshire Reference Works, 2002), 185–92.

22. L. Behl, H. Conyngham, and P. May, "Trends in Child Maltreatment Literature," *Child Abuse and Neglect* 27 (2002): 215–29.

23. B. D. Perry, K. Colwell, and S. Schick, "Child Neglect," in *Encyclopedia of Crime and Punishment,* vol. 1, ed. D. Levinson (Great Barrington, MA: Berkshire Reference Works, 2002), 192–96.

24. Table adapted from Drug Endangered Children (DEC), *Drug Endangered Children Health and Safety Manual.*

25. H. Dubowitz et al., "Child Neglect: Outcomes in High-Risk Urban Preschoolers," *Pediatrics* 109, no. 6 (2002): 1100–108.

26. M. D. Ainsworth et al., *Patterns of Attachment: A Psychological Study of the Strange Situation* (Hillsdale, NJ: Erlbaum, 1978); J. Bowlby, *A Secure Base: Clinical Application of Attachment Theory* (London: Routledge, 1988); M. Main, "Recent Studies in Attachment: Overview, with Selected Implications for Clinical Work," in *Attachment Theory: Social, Development, and Clinical Perspectives,* ed. S. Goldberg and R. Muir (Hillsdale, NJ: Analytic Press, 1995).

27. Dubowitz et al., "Child Neglect," 1100–108; Hildyard and Wolfe, "Child Neglect," 679–95; Perry, Colwell, and Schick, "Child Neglect," 192–96; A. Rosas, "Medical Diagnosis of Child Abuse and Neglect," in *Handbook for the Treatment of Child Maltreatment,* ed. F. Talley and A. Urquiza (Boston: Allyn and Bacon, in press).

28. Dubowitz et al., "Child Neglect," 1100–108.

29. Perry, Colwell, and Schick, "Child Neglect," 192–96; R. Pynoos et al., "Issues in the Developmental Neurobiology of Traumatic Stress," *Annals of the New York Academy of Sciences* 821 (1997): 176–93.

30. Dunn et al, "Origins and Consequences of Child Neglect," 1063–90; S. Thompson, "Working with Children of Substance-Abusing Parents," *Young Children* 53, no. 1 (1998): 34–37.

31. R. Dembo et al., "The Relationship between Physical and Sexual Abuse and Illicit Drug Use: A Replication among a New Sample of Youths Entering a Juvenile Detention Center," *International Journal of the Addictions* 23, no. 11 (1988): 1101–23; Hildyard and Wolfe, "Child Neglect," 679–95; S. Simon et al., "Methamphetamine Abuse: Associations with Early Academic Performance," *Journal of Addictive Diseases* 19, no. 2 (2000): 21.

32. S. Dube et al., "Childhood Abuse, Household Dysfunction, and the Risk of Attempted Suicide throughout the Life Span: Findings from the Adverse Childhood Experiences Study," *Journal of the American Medical Association* 286, no. 24 (2001): 3089–96; J. Stein, M. B. Leslie, and A. Nyamathi, "Relative Contributions of Parent Substance Use and Childhood Maltreatment to Chronic Homelessness, Depression, and Substance Abuse Problems among Homeless Women: Mediating Roles of Self-Esteem and Abuse in Adulthood," *Child Abuse and Neglect* 26, no. 10 (2002): 1011–27.

33. K. Brohl, *Working with Traumatized Children: A Handbook for Healing* (Washington, DC: CWLA Press, 1996); Hildyard and Wolfe, "Child Neglect," 679–95; S. Kang, S. Deren, and M. Goldstein, "Relationships between Childhood Abuse and Neglect Experience and HIV Risk Behaviours among Methadone Treatment Drop-Outs," *Child Abuse and Neglect* 26, no. 12 (2002): 1275–89.

34. Perry, Colwell, and Schick, "Child Neglect," 192–196; J. Wood et al., "An Examination of the Relationship between Violence Exposure, Post Traumatic Stress Symptomatology, and Delinquent Activity: An 'Ecopathological' Model of Delinquent Behavior among Incarcerated Adolescents," *Journal of Aggression, Maltreatment, and Trauma* 6, no. 1 (2002): 127–47.

35. Hildyard and Wolfe "Child Neglect," 679–95; J. T. Manly et al., "Dimensions of Child Maltreatment and Children's Adjustment: Contributions of Developmental Timing and Subtype," *Development and Psychopathology* 13 (2001): 759–82; Perry, Colwell, and Schick, "Child Neglect," 192–96; R. Pynoos, A. Steinberg, E. Ornitz, and A. Goenjian, "Issues in the Developmental Neurobiology of Traumatic Stress," *Annals of the New York Academy of Sciences* 821 (1997): 176–93.

36. K. Bolger and C. Patterson, "Developmental Pathways from Child Maltreatment to Peer Rejection," *Child Development* 69 (2001): 1171–97.

37. D. Wolfe and R. McGee, "Child Maltreatment and Adolescent Adjustment," *Development and Psychopathology* 6 (1994): 165–81.

38. Stein, Leslie, and Nyamathi, "Relative Contributions of Parent Substance Use," 1011–27.

39. R. Z. Dominguez, C. F. Nelke, and B. D. Perry, "Child Sexual Abuse," in *Encyclopedia of Crime and Punishment,* vol. 1, ed. D. Levinson (Great Barrington, MA: Berkshire Reference Works, 2002), 202–7; J. Wood et al., "Violence Exposure and PTSD among Delinquent Girls," *Journal of Aggression, Maltreatment, and Trauma* 6, no. 1 (2002): 109–26.

40. B. Bloom, M. Chesney-Lind, and B. Owen, *Women in California Prisons: Hidden Victims of the War on Drugs* (San Francisco, CA: Center on Juvenile and Criminal Justice, 1994); D. McClellan, D. Farabee, and B. Couch, "Early Victimization, Drug Use, and Criminality: A Comparison of Male and Female Prisoners," *Criminal Justice and Behavior* 24, no. 4 (1997): 455–76.

41. Center for Substance Abuse Prevention, *Children Witnessing Violence* (SAMHSA, 2001), http://preventionpathways.samhsa.gov/pdfs/fact_children.pdf.

42. Center for Substance Abuse Prevention. *Children Witnessing Violence and Substance Abuse* (Rockville, MD: Substance Abuse and Mental Health Services Administration's [SAMHSA] National Clearinghouse for Alcohol and Drug Information, 2000), DHHS pub. no. SMA 00-3449.

43. Drug Enforcement Agency, statistics, www.usdoj.gov/dea (2000).

44. J. Deleon, "Children's Witnessing of Adult Domestic Violence," *Journal of Interpersonal Violence* 4, no. 8 (1999): 839–70; R. Pynoos, A. Steinberg, and J. C. Peacetime, "A Developmental Psychopathology Model of Childhood Traumatic Stress and Intersection with Anxiety Disorders," *Society of Biological Psychiatry* 46, no. 11 (1999): 1542–54; M. Shepard, "How Child Welfare Workers Assess and Intervene around Issues of Domestic Violence," *Child Maltreatment* 4, no. 2 (1999): 148–57.

45. Deleon, "Children's Witnessing," 839–70; Stein, Leslie, and Nyamathi, "Relative Contributions of Parent Substance Use," 1011–27.

46. Drug Endangered Children (DEC), *Drug Endangered Children Health and Safety Manual.*

47. Hohman, Oliver, and Wright, "Methamphetamine Abuse."

REFERENCES AND SUGGESTED READINGS

Suggested Readings for Chapter 1: Methamphetamine 101: The Basics

Office of Applied Studies. *Results from the 2002 National Survey on Drug Use and Health: Summary of National Findings.* NHSDA Series H-22, DHHS Publication No. SMA 03–3836, 2003. Rockville, MD: Substance Abuse and Mental Health Services Administration, 2003.

Office of Applied Studies. *Treatment Episode Data Set (TEDS): 1992–2001. National Admissions to Substance Abuse Treatment Services.* DASIS Series: S-20, DHHS Publication No. SMA 03-3778. Rockville, MD: Substance Abuse and Mental Health Services Administration, 2003.

Office of National Drug Control Policy (ONDCP). *Drug Policy Information Clearinghouse.* Washington, DC: Office of National Drug Control Policy, 2003.

Office on Drugs and Crime (UNODC) United Nations International Drug Control Programme (UNDCP). *Global Illicit Drug Trends 2003.* New York: United Nations Publication, 2003.

Thompson, P. M., et al. "Structural Abnormalities in the Brains of Human Subjects Who Use Methamphetamine." *Journal of Neuroscience* 24, no. 26 (2004): 6028–36.

References and Suggested Readings for Chapter 3: Effective Treatment—It Can Happen: Combining Knowledge, Experience, and Wisdom

Clay, R. A. "Cocaine Treatment Suggests Model for Methamphetamine." *SAMHSA News* 8 (Fall 2002): 8–11.

DuPont, R. L., T. M. Mieczkowski, and R. A. Newel. *Drug Testing in Correctional Settings: Guidelines for Effective Use.* Center City, MN: Hazelden, 2005.

Miller, W. R., and S. Rollnick. *Motivational Interviewing: Preparing People to Change.* 2nd ed. New York: Guilford, 2002.

National Institute of Justice. "Methamphetamine Interagency Task Force—Final Report: Federal Advisory Committee." 2004. Available at www.ojp.usdoj.gov/nij/methintf/contents.html.

Obert, J., et al. "Treating Substance Use Disorders." In *Handbook of Addictive Disorders: A Practical Guide to Diagnosis and Treatment,* ed. Robert Holman Coombs. Hoboken, NJ: Wiley Publishers, 2003.

Obert, J. L., E. D. London, and R. A. Rawson. "Incorporating Brain Research Findings into Standard Treatment: An Example Using the Matrix Model." *Journal of Substance Abuse Treatment* 23 (2002): 107–14.

Obert, J. L., et al. "The Matrix Model of Outpatient Stimulant Abuse Treatment, History and Description." *Journal of Psychoactive Drugs* 32, no. 2 (2000): 157–64.

Prochaska, James O., John Norcross, and Carlo DiClemente. *Changing for Good.* New York: William Morrow and Company, Inc., 1994.

Washton, A. M., ed. *Psychotherapy and Substance Abuse: A Practitioner's Handbook.* New York: Guilford, 1995.

Suggested Readings for Chapter 5: Adolescents and Meth

California Department of Alcohol and Drug Treatment. *Youth Treatment Guidelines.* ADP Publication #8566. Sacramento, CA: California Department of Alcohol and Drug Treatment, 2002.

Center for Substance Abuse Treatment. "The Cannabis Youth Treatment (CYT) Experiment: Preliminary Findings." A report to H. Westley Clark, 2002.

Monti, P. M., S. M. Colby, T. A. O'Leary, eds. *Adolescents, Alcohol, and Substance Abuse.* New York: Guilford, 2001.

National Institute of Justice. "Methamphetamine Interagency Task Force—Final Report: Federal Advisory Committee." 2004. Available at www.ojp.usdoj.gov/nij/methintf/contents.html.

Obert, J. L., et al. "The Matrix Model of Outpatient Stimulant Abuse Treatment, History and Description." *Journal of Psychoactive Drugs* 32, no. 2 (2000): 157–64.

Sloboda, Z., and S. L. David. *Preventing Drug Use among Children and Adolescents.* NIH publication no. 04-4212A. Bethesda, MD: National Institute on Drug Abuse, 2003.

■ ■ ■

ABOUT THE AUTHORS

Jeanne L. Obert, M.F.T., M.S.M., is a founder and the executive director of Matrix Institute, an outpatient treatment center in the greater Los Angeles area, with five sites. She is the director of Outpatient Services for the Matrix/UCLA Integrated Substance Abuse Programs. Obert is a licensed marriage and family therapist and an AAMFT supervisor. She is a Motivational Interviewing (MI) trainer, originally trained by William Miller in 1993, and has done MI trainings in conjunction with Matrix Model workshops for many years. She originated and developed the clinical training programs at Matrix Institute and for the Center for Substance Abuse Treatment (CSAT)-funded national multisite study of the Matrix Model Methamphetamine Treatment Project. Recently, she served as an expert trainer on a Motivational Enhancement study being led by Yale University as part of the NIDA Clinical Trials Network (CTN), and presently she is the project director on a CSAT-funded study of effective adolescent treatment. Obert has performed trainings and consultations throughout the United States and internationally in Thailand, South Africa, Sweden, Israel, and Brazil. She has authored or co-authored more than fifty articles, book chapters, and treatment manuals. Several of the recent articles describing the Matrix Model of treatment explain how the model incorporates and uses recent research findings and elaborate on efforts to replicate the programs in community-based clinics.

Michael J. McCann, M.A., is one of the founders of the Matrix Institute and is the associate director and director of research. He has more than twenty-five years of experience in substance abuse treatment and research, and he has authored or co-authored more than thirty articles and books in the area, including a technical assistance publication for the Center for Substance Abuse Treatment (CSAT) on counseling in opioid treatment programs and an online course for counseling buprenorphine patients. He was the principal investigator for one of the sites in the Matrix Model Methamphetamine Treatment Project and also for the NIDA-funded Methamphetamine Clinical Trials Group. He is the project director for a CSAT-funded grant that is expanding treatment services for opioid dependence and providing evidence-based enhancements to standard services. McCann developed and implemented an outcomes management system in the Matrix clinics and assisted in its implementation in Thailand. He has developed and overseen the operation of Matrix clinics as well as the integration of many research projects within these sites. He has trained and lectured on outpatient treatment, behavioral interventions, pharmacologic treatments, and the implementation of research findings into clinical practice.

Patricia Marinelli-Casey, Ph.D., has been involved in substance abuse and mental health research and treatment since 1985. She is an assistant research psychologist at UCLA and serves as the principal investigator for three Center for Substance Abuse Treatment (CSAT)-funded studies focusing on methamphetamine. Marinelli-Casey's areas of expertise include methamphetamine treatment research, the implementation of pharmacotherapies in addiction treatment, substance abuse in the workplace, and the changing provision of substance abuse treatment and mental health services under managed care. Marinelli-Casey serves as an "addiction expert" for the Entertainment Industries Council and has provided numerous trainings and consultations on the "science of addiction." Prior to her current position at UCLA, Marinelli-Casey worked as a clinician providing direct care and as an administrator for various behavioral health care organizations. She served as the director of program development for Matrix Institute and as an employee assistance professional for the Entertainment Industry Referral and Assistance Center. Marinelli-Casey received her bachelor's degree in psychology from Santa Clara University, her master's degree in community/clinical psychology from California State University, Northridge (CSUN), and her doctorate in education from the University of California, Los Angeles (UCLA). Marinelli-Casey is a licensed marriage and family therapist (MFT) in the state of California.

Richard A. Rawson received a Ph.D. in experimental psychology from the University of Vermont in 1974. He has spent his career conducting research and developing systems for treating individuals with substance use disorders. Rawson has been a member of the UCLA department of psychiatry for more than twenty years and is currently an adjunct associate professor and the associate director of the UCLA Integrated Substance Abuse Programs. In this role, Rawson oversees a portfolio of addiction research ranging from brain imaging studies, to numerous clinical trials on pharmacological and psychosocial addiction treatments, to the study of how new treatments are applied in the treatment system. During the past decade, he has worked with the U.S. State Department on large substance abuse research and treatment projects, exporting U.S. technology and addiction science to Mexico, Thailand, Israel, Egypt, South Africa, and the Palestinian Authority. He is currently principal investigator of the Pacific Southwest Addiction Technology Transfer Center and the NIDA Methamphetamine Clinical Trials Group, and co-principal investigator of the Pacific Node of the NIDA Clinical Trials Network (CTN). Rawson has published 2 books, 20 book chapters, and more than 150 professional papers, and has conducted more than 1,000 workshops, paper presentations, and training sessions.

■ ■ ■

Hazelden Publishing and Educational Services is a division of the Hazelden Foundation, a not-for-profit organization. Since 1949, Hazelden has been a leader in promoting the dignity and treatment of people afflicted with the disease of chemical dependency.

The mission of the foundation is to improve the quality of life for individuals, families, and communities by providing a national continuum of information, education, and recovery services that are widely accessible; to advance the field through research and training; and to improve our quality and effectiveness through continuous improvement and innovation.

Stemming from that, the mission of this division is to provide quality information and support to people wherever they may be in their personal journey—from education and early intervention, through treatment and recovery, to personal and spiritual growth.

Although our treatment programs do not necessarily use everything Hazelden publishes, our bibliotherapeutic materials support our mission and the Twelve Step philosophy upon which it is based. We encourage your comments and feedback.

The headquarters of the Hazelden Foundation are in Center City, Minnesota. Additional treatment facilities are located in Chicago, Illinois; Newberg, Oregon; New York, New York; Plymouth, Minnesota; and St. Paul, Minnesota. At these sites, we provide a continuum of care for men and women of all ages. Our Plymouth facility is designed specifically for youth and families.

For more information on Hazelden, please call **1-800-257-7800.**

Or you may access our World Wide Web site on the Internet at **www.hazelden.org.**